Imaging Informatics for Healthcare Professionals

AF273262

Series Editors

Peter M. A. van Ooijen, University Medical Center Groningen,
University of Groningen, GRONINGEN, The Netherlands

Erik Ranschaert, Faculty of Medicine and Health Sciences,
Ghent University, Ghent, Belgium

Annalisa Trianni, Department of Medical Physics, ASUIUD,
UDINE, Italy

Michail E. Klontzas, Institute of Computer Science, Foundation
for Research and Technology (FORTH) and University Hospital
of Heraklion, Heraklion, Greece

The series Imaging Informatics for Healthcare Professionals is the ideal starting point for physicians and residents and students in radiology and nuclear medicine who wish to learn the basics in different areas of medical imaging informatics. Each volume is a short pocket-sized book that is designed for easy learning and reference.

The scope of the series is based on the Medical Imaging Informatics subsections of the European Society of Radiology (ESR) European Training Curriculum, as proposed by ESR and the European Society of Medical Imaging Informatics (EuSoMII). The series, which is endorsed by EuSoMII, will cover the curricula for Undergraduate Radiological Education and for the level I and II training programmes. The curriculum for the level III training programme will be covered at a later date. It will offer frequent updates as and when new topics arise.

Erik Ranschaert
Mohammad H. Rezazade Mehrizi
Willem Grootjans · Tessa S. Cook
Editors

AI Implementation in Radiology

Challenges and Opportunities in Clinical Practice

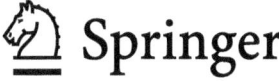 Springer

Editors
Erik Ranschaert
Faculty of Medicine and Health
Sciences
Ghent University
Ghent, Belgium

Willem Grootjans
Department of Radiology
Leiden University Medical Center
Leiden, The Netherlands

Mohammad H. Rezazade Mehrizi
School of Business and
Economics
Vrije Universiteit Amsterdam
Amsterdam, Noord-Holland,
The Netherlands

Tessa S. Cook
Department of Radiology
Hospital of University of
Pennsylvania
Philadelphia, PA, USA

ISSN 2662-1541　　　　　　　　ISSN 2662-155X　(electronic)
Imaging Informatics for Healthcare Professionals
ISBN 978-3-031-68941-3　　　　ISBN 978-3-031-68942-0　(eBook)
https://doi.org/10.1007/978-3-031-68942-0

This Springer imprint is published by the registered company Springer Nature Switzerland AG
The registered company address is: Gewerbestrasse 11, 6330 Cham, Switzerland

If disposing of this product, please recycle the paper.

Contents

1 **Introduction** 1
   Erik Ranschaert, Mohammad H. Rezazade Mehrizi,
   Willem Grootjans, and Tessa S. Cook

2 **Identification of the Need for Change** 11
   Willem Grootjans and Mark van Buchem

3 **Planning and Goal Setting** 33
   Elmar Kotter

4 **Stakeholder Engagement and Communication** 51
   Kayla Berigan, Tessa S. Cook, and Erik Ranschaert

5 **Exploring and Assessing AI Models** 69
   Peter M. A. van Ooijen and Sergey Morozov

6 **Legal and Ethical Aspects of AI in Radiology** 87
   Bart Custers and Eduard Fosch-Villaronga

7 **Workflow Integration and Training** 107
   João Abrantes and Willem Grootjans

8 **Evaluation, Monitoring, and Improvement** 131
   Willem Grootjans

9 **The Impact of AI on Radiology Reporting** 161
   J. M. Nobel

Introduction

Erik Ranschaert ⓘ,
Mohammad H. Rezazade Mehrizi,
Willem Grootjans ⓘ, and Tessa S. Cook ⓘ

> **Key Points**
> - Effective implementation and use of artificial intelligence (AI) in radiology require managing the process of change in technological landscape, clinical and non-clinical workflow, human roles and skills, and organisational structures and policies.

E. Ranschaert (✉)
Department of Radiology, St. Nikolaus Hospital, Eupen, Belgium

Faculty of Medicine and Health Sciences, Ghent University, Ghent, Belgium

M. H. Rezazade Mehrizi
School of Business and Economics, Vrije Universiteit Amsterdam, Amsterdam, The Netherlands
e-mail: m.rezazademehrizi@vu.nl

W. Grootjans
Department of Radiology, Leiden University Medical Center, Leiden, Zuid-Holland, The Netherlands
e-mail: w.grootjans@lumc.nl

T. S. Cook
Department of Radiology, University of Pennsylvania, Philadelphia, PA, USA
e-mail: Tessa.Cook@pennmedicine.upenn.edu

- The change management process demands an on-going set of essential activities such as identification of the needs (for change), planning and goal setting, engaging stakeholders, exploring and assessing the AI solutions, arranging for legal and ethical aspects, integrating AI solutions into the workflow and training users, and continuous evaluation and improvement.
- The results of such change management must be clearly linked to strategic and operational goals of medical institutions and be effectively realised along the change management process.

1.1 Introduction

There is no denying that more and more radiology departments are implementing AI applications to enhance and streamline various tasks within their workflows. The number of commercially available and thus certified AI products is already impressive, and both the number and variety of applications continue to grow steadily. As a result, AI will not only transform clinical practice but also the organisation and management of the entire radiology department. Indeed, the use of AI technology requires entirely new policies within the radiology department, because of its impact on many different parts of the radiology workflow, and even beyond. The scope of this impact is something that is often underestimated in practice, or of which radiology staff and other healthcare professionals are not fully aware. However, the successful implementation of AI applications relies on a well-coordinated multidisciplinary effort to ensure their optimal integration and safe, effective, use. The purpose of this book is to provide practical insights and offer guidance on how to successfully adopt AI applications in clinical practice.

The integration of AI applications in radiology offers numerous advantages and exciting possibilities for improved patient care and workflow optimisation and improving quality of radiological services delivered [1]. Moreover, AI applications can greatly help in workload management, not only by automating routine tasks, such as image analysis, but even report generation [2]. This digital assistance brings about new forms of collaboration between humans and technology that can lead to a shift in roles and responsibilities between different radiology professionals supported by AI technology [3]. Such a hybrid partnership between humans and AI allows radiology professionals to build on their expertise by leveraging the information provided by AI applications, thereby adding new data to the radiological report that may not have been available before. In particular, the integration of quantitative data improves disease characterisation for better diagnosis and clinical decision-making. Moreover, automating image analysis tasks frees up time for radiologists and reporting radiographers to use their expertise for more complex cases, potentially increasing the overall productivity and reducing turnaround times [4]. Through automated generation of results and considering patient specific medical history and conditions, the use of AI has the capability to facilitate personalised medicine by tailoring treatment plans. This personalised approach can lead to more effective and targeted treatments, ultimately benefiting both patients and healthcare providers [5].

Despite the promising benefits, the implementation of AI in radiology also brings a number of challenges, which also require making the necessary changes not only at the departmental but also hospital-wide level. An AI implementation process usually starts with assessing the existing difficulties in the workflow, for which an appropriate AI software and hardware solution could be searched, aligning with the uniquely identified needs of the department and or medical institution. This is inevitably followed by ensuring the interoperability with existing IT-systems within the department and the medical institution [6–8]. Consecutively, radiology departments might need to undergo several changes in management strategies to facilitate the integration of one or more different AI solutions. This is mainly because the integration of AI technology is less about fitting a particular new application into an existing environment as it is about realignment and modifying all the related components in the workflow, technical infrastructure, as well as roles and responsibilities, culture, and expertise of involved professionals. The ultimate goal of these changes would be to improve the radiology services to referring physicians and patients, as well as enriching the work of radiology professionals and improving their working experience with the assistance of AI. Therefore, the precise goals and expectations need to be defined as well. These requirements make the integration of AI technology a complex process that involves careful goal setting and planning, which will be discussed in detail in Chaps. 2 and 3.

Chapters 2 and 3 focus on the different components and steps of the implementation process of AI technology in the radiological and clinical environment, explaining the importance of first assessing the existing situation so that the best use-cases can be defined for selecting an AI-based application and for setting the appropriate goals to be reached.

The processes and changes related to the implementation of AI in radiological practice often go beyond the radiology department and implicate other medical domains and departments with which radiologists collaborate. This means it is necessary to engage other stakeholders in the implementation process, which requires setting up an organisational infrastructure. Ideally, a team involving all decision-making parties should be created to streamline the entire process as much as possible. The team can consist not only of permanent members, but also of internal or external consultants, who can also be consulted as needed. The members of this team are mainly to be sought from other parts of the hospital such as the IT department, the PACS managers, the procurement department, the data privacy officer (DPO), the Chief Medical Information Officer (CMIO), the referring clinicians, the persons responsible for training, the medical council, and the board of directors, among others [9, 10]. In addition, engaging referring physicians and other medical specialities that will use radiological reports for clinical decision-making is crucial to ensure that changes are aligned with the final medical services to be delivered.

Chapter 4 addresses the need for involving various stakeholders both inside and outside the radiology department, as well as their role in the proper and safe implementation of AI in radiological practice.

Once the basic infrastructure is formed, the consultation team can look at which applications qualify for a specific use case, and how these existing commercial models can be evaluated. The team can set up a system that uses specific objectives or Key Performance Indicators (KPIs) to check whether or not a commercially available solution meets the predefined expectations and requirements. These requirements should be seen broadly and cannot be limited to the clinical applicability. Of course, it is also about integrability with existing systems, and the continuous monitoring of performance and quality of the solution(s) once implemented. All these topics are discussed further in Chap. 5.

Chapter 5 looks at how to assess what AI-based solutions are available, and how they can be evaluated, validated, and finally integrated into the local system(s). Various methods of monitoring the performance and reliability of these devices, both technically and clinically are also discussed.

When it comes to the formal aspects, developing a robust data governance framework is also essential to handle patient data securely and responsibly, addressing concerns related to privacy and security [11]. Before implementing AI applications, it is necessary to inform and consult the existing bodies in the hospital for this purpose, so that the appropriate contracts are concluded, in accordance with the existing regulations and legislature. The medical ethics committee must also approve the way in which patient data are processed and used. It is very important to pay attention to the various contractual agreements that need to be concluded between the vendors and healthcare providers or hospitals on the one hand, and the expertise and internal decisions required for that purpose [7, 12, 13].

Chapter 6 is focusing on different contractual agreements, including the regulatory and ethical issues that are relevant when using AI technology in radiology.

For effective implementation and use, collaboration between radiology professionals and AI systems plays a pivotal role in achieving successful safe and effective use. Therefore, radiology professionals should gain a comprehensive understanding of the strengths and limitations of AI models and actively participate in their validation and fine-tuning to enhance performance continually [7, 9, 10]. This requires radiology department management to optimally redistribute tasks amongst different professionals by facilitating the creation of new roles and responsibilities. New functions will be added consisting of overseeing the correct implementation of available AI systems and validating their outputs. A group-wide vision must be formed about analysing, reporting, and storing the AI results. As such, department leaders must foster a culture of continuous learning and innovation, encouraging staff members to embrace AI technologies as valuable tools in their practice without being seen as added work on already overextended physicians. To ensure smooth adoption of AI in radiology departments, comprehensive training programs should be provided for radiologists, radiographers, and radiology residents. These programs will help users to develop the necessary skills to effectively and safely work with AI technology [14].

All facets related to the changing roles of radiologists and the impact of AI on training, evaluation, and monitoring will be addressed in Chaps. 7 and 8.

Chapters 7 and 8 cover the changing roles of radiologists, the impact of AI on training, evaluation, and monitoring, as well as the necessity for collaboration between radiology professionals and AI systems in the course of performing clinical tasks.

Although deep learning techniques, specifically convolutional neural networks (CNNs), have been widely used for various imaging tasks in radiology, such as image classification and segmentation, newer AI technologies like generative AI and large language models (LLMs) are beginning to find applications in the field. These might be used for tasks such as generating synthetic medical images for training or research, enhancing image resolution, or extracting and synthesising information from radiological reports. These AI technologies will affect the way digital reports are generated, which is currently largely done using speech recognition. With these new generative models, highly efficient, assistive solutions for information management and report generation might be developed. Such applications could significantly transform data management workflows in radiology and more generally in healthcare and medicine. There is no denying that they may soon have a significant impact on the way radiological reports are made, as well as on the form and content of these reports [2, 15, 16]. The possibilities and possible impact of these new techniques on radiology reporting will be addressed in Chap. 9.

Chapter 9 discusses the emerging deep learning techniques and their potential impact on radiological report generation.

This book is the result of collaboration between leading experts in their fields, combining practical wisdom and scientific acumen. It was our intention to convey our insights to you, the reader, in a bundled and structured manner, so that you can get started with them in your clinical practice. Thus, in the chapters that follow, you should be able to find the most relevant information on challenges you may face in a practical implementation process of AI applications in your clinical environment. However, it is important to recognise that while we have strived to cover a broad spectrum of insights, it was not easy to cover every facet of change management comprehensively in these pages. In fact, many devils of change management are in the details that must be experienced and worked out in each and every individual case of AI implementation.

1.2   Conclusion

In this book, we delve into the profound impact of AI integration in radiology. We explore how AI technologies are poised to enhance diagnostic accuracy, streamline workflows, and improve patient outcomes. Furthermore, we examine the challenges and opportunities associated with this transformative shift, offering insights and guidance on how radiology departments can successfully adapt to this new era of radiological practice. With each chapter, we will elaborate on separate management issues and try to give you a better understanding of the changes and adaptations involved in the application of AI in clinical practice.

References

1. Hosny A, Parmar C, Quackenbush J, Schwartz LH, Aerts HJWL. Artificial intelligence in radiology. Nat Rev Cancer. 2018;18:500–10. https://doi.org/10.1038/s41568-018-0016-5.

2. D'Antonoli TA, Stanzione A, Bluethgen C, Vernuccio F, Ugga L, Klontzas ME, Cuocolo R, Cannella R, Koçak B. Large language models in radiology: fundamentals, applications, ethical considerations, risks, and future directions. Diagn Interv Radiol. 2023;30:80–90. https://doi.org/10.4274/dir.2023.232417.

3. Mehrizi MHR. Pre-framing an emerging technology before it is deployed at work: the case of artificial intelligence and radiology. J Comput-Mediat Commun. 2023;28:zmad029. https://doi.org/10.1093/jcmc/zmad029.

4. Ranschaert E, Topff L, Pianykh O. Optimization of radiology workflow with artificial intelligence. Radiol Clin N Am. 2021;59:955–66. https://doi.org/10.1016/j.rcl.2021.06.006.

5. Steyaert S, Pizurica M, Nagaraj D, Khandelwal P, Hernandez-Boussard T, Gentles AJ, Gevaert O. Multimodal data fusion for cancer biomarker discovery with deep learning. Nat Mach Intell. 2023;5:351–62. https://doi.org/10.1038/s42256-023-00633-5.

6. Omoumi P, Ducarouge A, Tournier A, Harvey H, Kahn CE, Verchère FL, Santos DPD, Kober T, Richiardi J. To buy or not to buy—evaluating commercial AI solutions in radiology (the ECLAIR guidelines). Eur Radiol. 2021;31:3786–96. https://doi.org/10.1007/s00330-020-07684-x.

7. Daye D, Wiggins WF, Lungren MP, Alkasab T, Kottler N, Allen B, Roth CJ, Bizzo BC, Durniak K, Brink JA, Larson DB, Dreyer KJ, Langlotz CP. Implementation of clinical artificial intelligence in radiology: who decides and how? Radiology. 2022;305:555–63. https://doi.org/10.1148/radiol.212151.

8. Strohm L, Hehakaya C, Ranschaert ER, Boon WPC, Moors EHM. Implementation of artificial intelligence (AI) applications in radiology: hindering and facilitating factors. Eur Radiol. 2020;1–8 https://doi.org/10.1007/s00330-020-06946-y.

9. Rubin DL. Artificial intelligence in imaging: the radiologist's role. J Am Coll Radiol. 2019;16:1309–17. https://doi.org/10.1016/j.jacr.2019.05.036.

10. Kotter E, Ranschaert E. Challenges and solutions for introducing artificial intelligence (AI) in daily clinical workflow. Eur Radiol. 2021;31:1–3. https://doi.org/10.1007/s00330-020-07148-2.

11. Murdoch B. Privacy and artificial intelligence: challenges for protecting health information in a new era. Bmc Med Ethics. 2021;22:122. https://doi.org/10.1186/s12910-021-00687-3.

12. European Society of Radiology (ESR). The new EU general data protection regulation: what the radiologist should know. Insights Imaging. 2017;8:295–9. https://doi.org/10.1007/s13244-017-0552-7.

13. Liew C. The future of radiology augmented with artificial intelligence: a strategy for success. Eur J Radiol. 2018;102:152–6. https://doi.org/10.1016/j.ejrad.2018.03.019.

14. Wiggins WF, Caton MT, Magudia K, Glomski SA, George E, Rosenthal MH, Gaviola GC, Andriole KP. Preparing radiologists to lead in the era of

artificial intelligence: designing and implementing a focused data science pathway for senior radiology residents. Radiology Artif Intell. 2020;2:e200057. https://doi.org/10.1148/ryai.2020200057.

15. Alayrac J-B, Donahue J, Luc P, Miech A, Barr I, Hasson Y, Lenc K, Mensch A, Millican K, Reynolds M, Ring R, Rutherford E, Cabi S, Han T, Gong Z, Samangooei S, Monteiro M, Menick J, Borgeaud S, Brock A, Nematzadeh A, Sharifzadeh S, Binkowski M, Barreira R, Vinyals O, Zisserman A, Simonyan K. Flamingo: a visual language model for few-shot learning. arXiv. 2023; https://doi.org/10.48550/arxiv.2204.14198.

16. Harrer S. Attention is not all you need: the complicated case of ethically using large language models in healthcare and medicine. Ebiomedicine. 2023;90:104512. https://doi.org/10.1016/j.ebiom.2023.104512.

Identification of the Need for Change

2

Willem Grootjans and Mark van Buchem

> **Key Points**
> - Over the years, radiology has acquired a central role in healthcare.
> - The success of radiology has resulted in increased imaging demands and workload in the radiology department.
> - Successful use of AI in radiology requires a holistic implementation strategy.
> - The use of AI can add significant value to the radiology value chain, improving efficiency and patient care.
> - Embracing AI in radiology necessitates process re-evaluation and ongoing adaptation.

2.1 A Success Story with a Dark Side

Since the discovery of the X-rays by Wilhelm Conrad Röntgen in 1895, the field of radiology has had a major impact on clinical medicine. Continuous technological development has led to the

W. Grootjans (✉) · M. van Buchem
Department of Radiology, Leiden University Medical Center, Leiden, Zuid-Holland, The Netherlands
e-mail: w.grootjans@lumc.nl; m.a.van_buchem@lumc.nl

© The Author(s), under exclusive license to Springer Nature Switzerland AG 2024
E. Ranschaert et al. (eds.), *AI Implementation in Radiology*, Imaging Informatics for Healthcare Professionals,
https://doi.org/10.1007/978-3-031-68942-0_2

availability of a wealth of imaging techniques allowing for non-invasive detection, visualisation, and characterisation of internal anatomy and pathology in patients. The relevance of this information for clinical practice has led to a rapid increase in the use of radiological services, with an estimated annual growth rate of 5–10% for decades in a row [1–4]. As a result, radiology has acquired a central role in healthcare [5]. Apart from the introduction of new imaging techniques, radiology was the first field in medicine where digitisation was introduced on a large scale, during the last decade of the twentieth century. The advent of digital radiology marked a pivotal moment, where analogue films gave way to digital images, making storage, retrieval, and transmission of radiological data more efficient. This transition accelerated the development of the Picture Archiving and Communication Systems (PACS), enabling electronic access to images throughout the hospital [6]. PACS has major logistical advantages: radiological images are always and instantly available on computers throughout a hospital system, whereas in the past, single cut films were generated that were available in only one place at a time and that often would get lost and had to be searched for. However, a major drawback of PACS is the reduced interaction between radiologists and referring physicians. Before the introduction of PACS, images and imaging experts were co-located in radiology departments, which stimulated interaction between referring physicians and radiologists. Based on such interactions, indications for imaging studies and the relevance and consequences of imaging findings were discussed. With PACS, such discussions have become less frequent which has affected the optimal use of imaging studies and contributed to increase in healthcare costs and unnecessary exposure to ionising irradiation in patients.

In addition to a steady annual growth, complexity of imaging studies themselves has increased. Conventional two-dimensional X-ray images with two projections have been replaced by three-dimensional tomographic studies, generating hundreds of images per study, considerably increasing the time radiologists spend on the interpretation of imaging studies. Furthermore, whereas radiologists previously relied solely on visual inspection of images, an array of advanced image processing tools has become available. These tools can be used for additional image analysis, yielding valuable quantitative information on patient physiology and disease state. Such quantitative assessments are relevant allowing for more objective and precise measurements of various physical properties and physiological processes of tissues, enabling improved diagnostic accuracy, monitoring of disease progression, and treatment planning [7]. Quantitative reporting not only enhances the consistency and reproducibility of radiological assessments but also opens the door to more robust research and the development of personalised treatment strategies. However, the introduction of quantitative analysis of medical images in clinical routine inevitably led to increased complexity, longer reporting times and therefore increased workload.

Increased workload has been a subject of discussion in the field of radiology for some time and is currently considered the biggest challenge in radiology. The increased radiological consumption and complexity of imaging studies have not been matched by a sufficiently increased workforce. This is reflected in the estimated prevalence of burnout among radiologists [8, 9], ranging between 33 and 88% [10], which is particularly high. The high workload, characterised by high caseloads and a continuous influx of images to interpret, often leads to long working hours, which can strain work-life balance. Radiologists also face the pressure of delivering accurate and timely reports, as their findings have a critical impact on patient care. Furthermore, the extensive use of technology and the expectation of rapid adaptation to new software tools also contributes to stress. Additionally, due to the PACS-based decreased interaction between radiologists and referring physicians, radiologists feel overworked, isolated and remote from patient care [10]. The cumulative effects of these stressors can result in emotional exhaustion, depersonalisation, and a diminished sense of personal accomplishment, all hallmark features of burnout. Similar trends in occupational burnout have been reported among radiographers and sonographers [11]. These professionals are facing high patient volumes, tight schedules, and the pressure to produce high-quality images, leading to physically and mentally demanding workdays. Additionally, the rapidly advancing technology in medical imaging requires continuous learning and adaptation, adding to the workload and stress. Therefore, it is of no surprise that addressing the causes of burnout in radiology and implementing strategies to support well-being of personnel is becoming increasingly important to maintain high-quality patient care and the overall sustainability of the field.

2.2 The Radiology Value Chain and AI

2.2.1 Supporting the Value Chain

Modern healthcare organisations are increasingly looking for innovative ways to redesign healthcare systems to ensure sustainable healthcare delivery [12, 13]. With rising costs and public expectations for continued delivery of high-quality care, there is an urgent need to balance the currently observed rise in healthcare expenditure [14]. The Institute for Healthcare Improvement (IHI) introduced the triple aim framework with three core goals: improving the experience of care, improving population health, and reducing per capita costs [15]. However, keeping current healthcare providers in the system and recruiting new providers have become a major challenge for the healthcare system. In recognition of this challenge, the triple aim has gradually been transformed into the quadruple aim, with improving healthcare provider satisfaction as a new dimension [16].

Translating the quadruple aim into the field of radiology, it is important to first define what radiology represents and how it adds value to healthcare. To this end, the concept of the value chain of radiology has been introduced and embraced by the American College of Radiology (ACR). This chain refers to the series of interconnected activities and processes involved in delivering radiological services [17]. It comprises the following stages: image ordering, acquisition and preprocessing, image analysis, image interpretation and reporting, communication, patient tracking and follow-up, quality assurance, research and education, administrative and operational support, patient care, and safety.

Over the years, several change initiatives have been proposed and implemented to increase the value of different components of the radiology value chain. From all these initiatives and technologies, artificial intelligence (AI) has recently generated high expectations to alleviate the burden on radiology departments [18]. Indeed, many consider the advent of AI as essential to ensure the sustainability of future radiology services, as it has the potential to elevate quality, enhance efficiency, and reduce the cost per radiological examination. While the concepts of modern AI technology can be traced back as far as the mid-50 s of the last century, the latest surge in interest emerged with the introduction of deep learning technologies in the mid-2010s [19]. It is important to recognise that AI is a broad-term encompassing various technologies that have been introduced over the years. In the context of modern radiology, the mention of AI typically refers to deep learning techniques. Deep learning techniques, particularly convolutional neural networks (CNNs), marked a turning point when such methods began to demonstrate remarkable success in tasks such as pattern recognition and segmentation, which are essential in many radiological applications [18, 20]. The main advantage of AI technology is that it offers remarkable flexibility and can be used for all stages of the radiological value chain and help contributing to achieving the quadruple aim [21]. For example, there are AI applications that can assist in image acquisition, reconstruction, optimising image quality, and reducing radiation exposure. Furthermore, AI-based applications can efficiently triage and prioritise cases, ensuring that urgent or critical studies receive prompt attention. In the interpretation phase, AI aids radiologists by rapidly identifying abnormalities, enhancing efficiency, and reducing the risk of oversight. Moreover, AI can play a crucial role in automating routine tasks such as annotation and image segmentation, and reporting, freeing up radiologists' time for more complex decision-making and patient interaction. Its versatility further extends to research and quality assurance, providing the basis of automated monitoring systems and acceleration of the development of new technology. Figure 2.1 depicts a typical radiological workflow, indicating areas where AI can provide assistance.

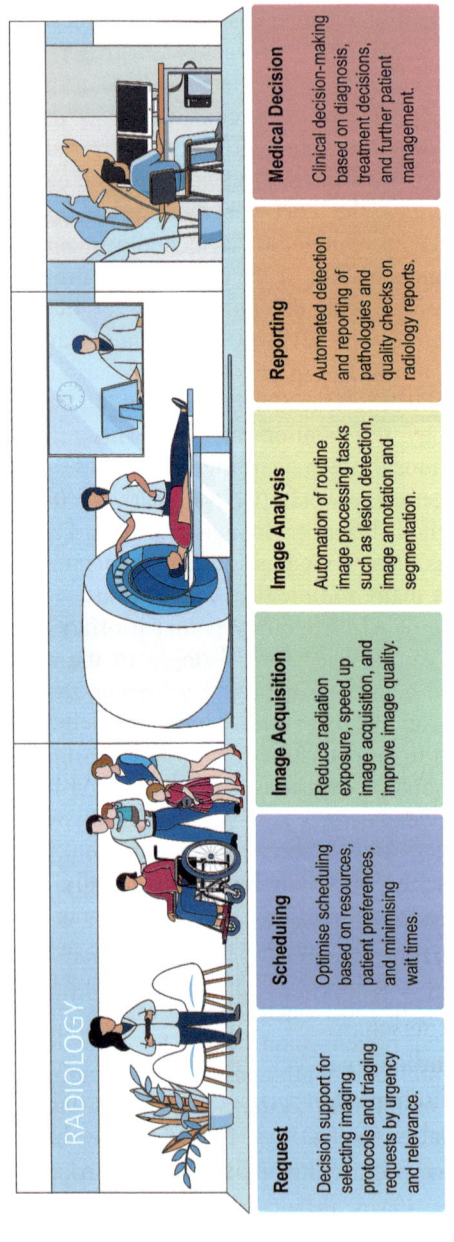

Fig. 2.1 Radiology value chain enhanced with artificial intelligence (AI) technology. There are several activities in the radiological workflow that can be enhanced with AI applications, focusing on improved efficiency and quality of radiological services delivered

2.2.2 Orchestration and Integration

While AI holds the potential to contribute across all parts of the radiology value chain, its widespread adoption in radiology departments around the world remains limited [22]. The current paradox, characterised by high expectations contrasted with the limited added value in existing workflows, hinders widespread implementation. In particular, as AI is currently an expensive technology, there is typically limited evidence supporting the claim of delivering systematic value to clinical practice [23]. Despite the creation and validation of numerous AI models through scientific studies, sustainable integration of AI applications into radiological workflows necessitates a comprehensive implementation of organisational and technological changes within the radiology department and, potentially, the entire hospital infrastructure. Even though AI applications, once integrated, can bring value to the clinical workflow, a challenge lies in their inherent specificity or narrow focus [24]. Hence, to maximise the benefits of AI technologies, it is necessary to employ multiple AI applications independently or utilise a sequential approach with different AI models to achieve meaningful workflow automation in clinical practice. This requires a technical infrastructure capable of orchestrating the complex routing of information and the transfer of both imaging and clinical data. Furthermore, the integration of AI-generated results into clinical front-end software systems such as PACS and advanced viewers is an ongoing development. The significance of seamless integrations has been underscored over the years, emphasising the need for minimal disruptions to the clinical workflow to facilitate the acceptance of AI by the radiology community.

2.2.3 Portfolio Management, Benefits, and Costs

In addition to achieving seamless integration of AI applications in clinical front-end systems and the meticulous routing and orchestration of their use within the clinical workflow, there is a need for active management of the portfolio of AI applications. While the combined use of multiple AI applications holds significant potential for delivering value, medical institutions often grapple with the question of which combination of applications will yield the most value for their practices. Furthermore, it is important to recognise the differences between institutions, there is not a one-size-fits-all optimal portfolio of AI applications for enhancing radiological workflows; instead, each institution will require a unique set of AI applications. Creating an effective AI portfolio requires in-depth insights into production metrics, workflow inefficiencies, and constraints. This insight will support a well-defined value proposition of specific AI applications (e.g. anticipated time reduction during reporting) that will result in a plan for return on investment. Radiology departments commonly face challenges in building a 'positive business case' for investing in AI technology. While small investment budgets are often allocated for rapid evaluation and experimentation of AI technology, these initiatives frequently do not lead to sustained use in radiological practice.

Moreover, the evaluation of radiology AI applications often relies on metrics confined to the radiology department, such as reduced reporting time, improving diagnosis and radiology service quality, decreased scan time, and improved radiologists' working experience. However, the broader impact of this technology across the entire healthcare chain is seldomly discussed. Involving other medical specialties in the integration of AI in radiology is imperative, as AI technology may have a more significant impact elsewhere in the healthcare chain than in radiology alone. For example, image segmentation might not only be of interest for the department of radiology, but also for the department of radiation oncology for the purpose of dosimetry and treatment planning. This could potentially open-up discussions about reallocating and sharing resources between departments to implement and maintain the use of AI technology within a healthcare institution. Equally important for the widespread adoption of AI in healthcare is the requirement for a fundamental shift in the financial system, including dedicated reimbursements for the use of AI technologies. While some countries have initiated initial efforts in this direction, there remains a critical need to reform healthcare systems to financially support adoption of AI technology into hospitals and healthcare practices [25]. However, careful design of payment for AI is essential for improving patient outcomes while maximising cost-effectiveness and equity [25]. With that being said, it is important to constantly re-evaluate the initial AI portfolio and continuously monitor its performance and added value, even after it's implementation. Regularly reassessing the portfolio to align with emerging trends and adapting strategies accordingly is crucial for long-term success in AI investment and portfolio management.

2.2.4   Return on Investment: The J-Curve

It is important to recognise that the adoption of AI involves an initial investment for the implementation phase to be made before realising any benefits. Initially, investments in personnel, software licences, and IT infrastructure may exceed the benefits derived from AI. However, with time, the advantages offered by AI should gradually offset this initial investment phase, resulting in positive outcomes. There is a strong parallel with the so-called J-curve of productivity, a well-known pattern seen in the adoption of new technology [26, 27]. The J-curve of productivity is a graphical representation of an investment's performance over time, characterised by an initial dip into negative values followed by a subsequent recovery to increasingly positive values, creating a pattern reminiscent of the letter 'J,' as illustrated in Fig. 2.2. It is worth noting that the trajectory of this initial investment can be initially disappointing, leading to a perception that AI has failed to deliver expected results. This perception is partly due to the fact that the anticipated cost savings, contingent on the specifics of a medical institution's financial system, may not materialise immediately.

Many departments experience that the required initial investment in AI technology is often underestimated. One of the foremost reasons for this is that the technology itself has not fully matured yet and AI applications are not simple plug-and-play solutions. Instead, they usually require significant customisation in order to be integrated into clinical practice. This means that the department or medical institution usually needs to allocate resources (personnel, hardware) to start hosting and integrating

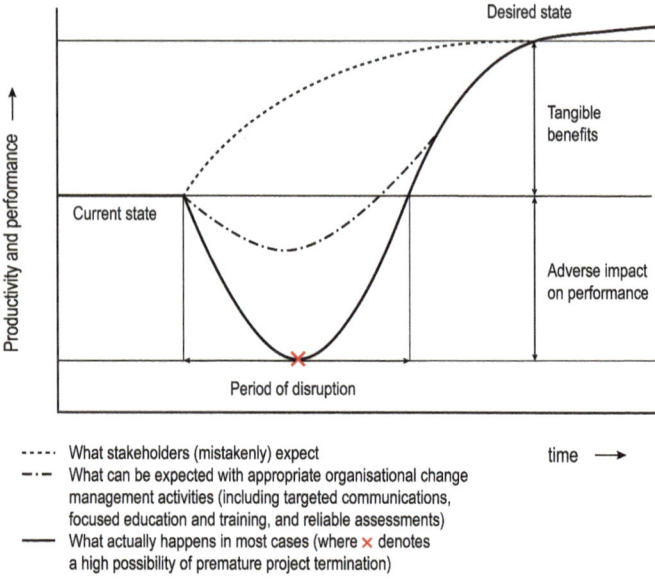

Fig. 2.2 The J-curve of change showing the initial performance of the implementation of new technology (including artificial intelligence (AI)). After initial implementation of an AI application, productivity and performance can significantly drop (also known as the period of disruption). Depending on how well the change management activities are organised, the depth of this initial disruption and thereby adverse impact may be mitigated. It is important to take stakeholder expectations into account, that might mistakenly expect a new innovation to yield tangible effects directly after implementation. Depending on the organisation's experience with technological implementation, the period of disruption might vary and be subjected to change over time, where more experienced organisations may have shorter disruption times than others. (Adapted from David Viney, the J-curve effect observed during change)

AI applications [22]. Although often overlooked, customisation and seamless integration of AI applications are not trivial and require significant efforts from both the radiology department or medical institution and the AI vendor. Reaching a seamless integration of AI applications in clinical front-end systems, such as PACS viewers or third-party software packages, is one of the key determinants in realising a tangible benefit for most AI applications. Disruptions caused by suboptimal integrations can quickly render an AI application ineffective and even counterproductive to use. In addition to the required resources for AI integrations, it is crucial that users receive adequate training to utilise new AI technology, making its use standard practice rather than optional and ensuring synchronised adoption in clinical settings. Maximising the tangible benefits from AI requires investing in comprehensive training programs and active expectation management [22].

Due to the substantial initial investment, the period of recovery can be significantly longer than expected or not be reached at all. The initial business case of specific AI applications is therefore of utmost importance to determine whether obtaining specific AI applications are beneficial. This is in turn closely related to the strategic goals and objectives of both the department and medical institution. In addition to the initial investments, it is important to consider the ongoing operational costs of AI. These operational costs are related to the use of specific resources (hardware, personnel) as well as licence fees for AI applications. Licence fees constitute a significant portion of the operational expenses, particularly when scaling the use of AI applications, often necessitating contractual agreements with various vendors. While licence models may vary, it is common to start from a base fee along with additional charges based on the volume of cases processed by the AI applications. Consequently, the realisation of benefits from AI may only occur after reaching a minimum volume of cases. These factors will ultimately determine the absolute benefit derived from AI and determine the timeframe for reaching a break-even point post-investment.

2.2.5 Technology Adoption: The S-Curve and Beyond

While the initial investment required for AI technology may indeed pose a considerable obstacle for radiology departments, the reluctance, fear, or resistance among professionals involved can represent a significant secondary barrier to its adoption and acceptance [28, 29]. Therefore, gaining insights into the dynamics surrounding the adoption of AI technology can assist department management to organise targeted change initiatives that facilitate its successful integration of AI applications. Everett Rogers' diffusion of innovation theory, which delineates the technology adoption lifecycle, provides a widely recognised framework for understanding the uptake of novel innovations [30]. The technology adoption life cycle acknowledges three distinct phases characterised by different user types. According to Rogers, the adoption of technology starts with innovators and early adopters, followed by an early and late majority, and concludes with laggards. The early and late majority users form the largest segment of the community, whereas early adopters and laggards constitute only a small percentage of total users, where the adoption of a new innovation by the community often adheres to a characteristic S-curve, as illustrated in Fig. 2.3.

Following Rogers' model, the current use of AI applications in radiology is primarily confined to early adopters. Therefore, facilitating the adoption of AI technology by the early and late majority of users is essential to increase acceptance of the technology and derive tangible benefits from broader utilisation. In order to do this, department management should provide targeted change initiatives that help facilitate the sociotechnical transitions that need to be made [22]. However, despite Rogers' diffusion of innovation theory providing a valuable framework for understanding technology adoption, its applicability may be limited when considering the unique complexities and dynamics of innovation adoption. This is particularly the case when studying the adoption of AI technology, characterised by many different stakeholders, complex decision-making processes, longer implementation timelines, and a strong interdependence of AI technology adoption with other organisational and technical innovations [31]. Therefore, Rogers' model of the technology adoption lifecycle is often complemented with other theoretical perspectives, such as the Normalisation Process Theory (NPT), described by May and colleagues, to achieve a more comprehensive understanding of healthcare innovation adoption processes [32, 33]. The strength of NPT lies in considering the cognitive and behavioural work individuals and groups undertake when integrating complex interventions into their social context, as illustrated in Fig. 2.4 [33].

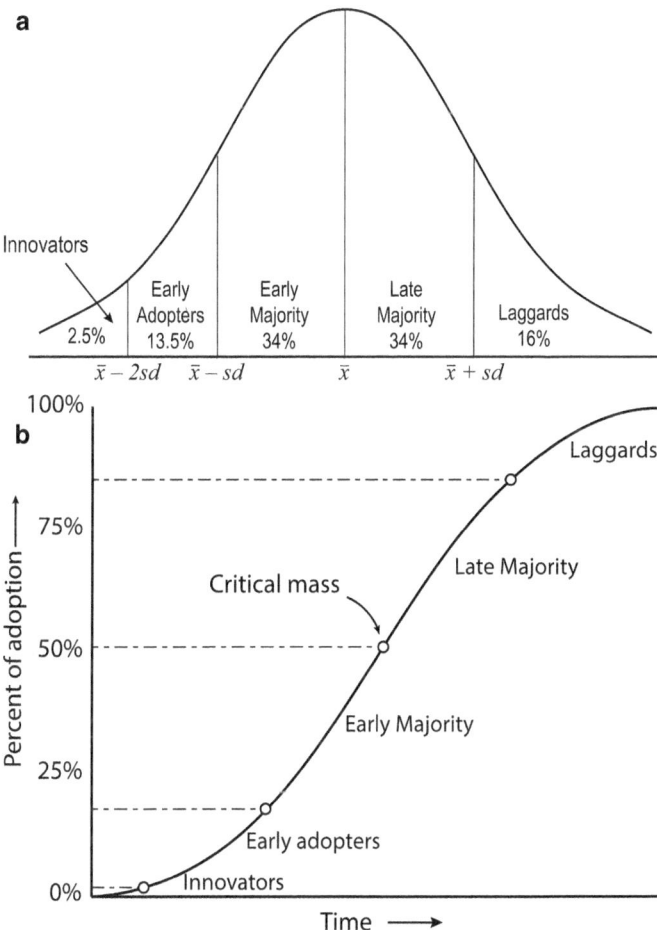

Fig. 2.3 Diffusion of innovation theory as proposed by Rogers. In this framework, adopters of technology are categorised into five segments (innovators, early adopters, early majority, late majority, and laggards). The contribution of each segment to the total community follows a normalised Gaussian distribution (**a**). The adoption of an innovation will gradually start with the innovators and early adopters, followed by the early majority (**b**). After adoption of an innovation by the early majority, a critical mass of users will have adopted the innovation and the process of further adoption will be self-sustaining. Roger's framework provides a basic understanding on the adoption of AI technology in the radiology community

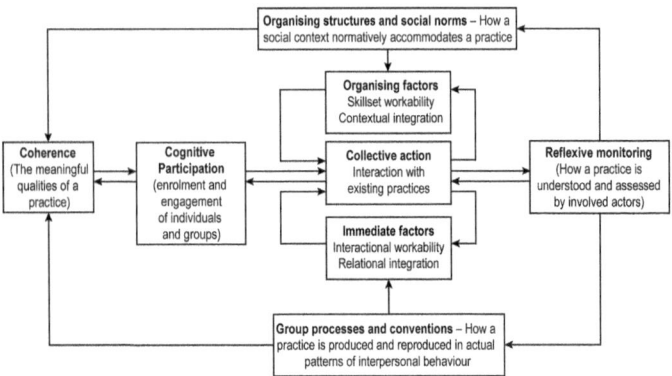

Fig. 2.4 Model of the components of normalisation process theory (NPT). The NTP model describes the interaction between four different components, namely coherence, cognitive participation, collective action, and reflexive monitoring. (Adapted from May et al. [33])

The four essential components of the NPT are coherence, cognitive participation, collective action, and reflexive monitoring [33]. Coherence refers to the establishment of a shared understanding of a practice within a community. It involves defining and organising the components of the practice, as well as investing meaning in it collectively. In the context of implementing AI in radiology, coherence would involve defining the roles and processes associated with AI integration, ensuring that all stakeholders understand and align with these definitions. Cognitive participation involves the engagement and enrolment of actors in the practice. It encompasses the initiation, enrolment, and legitimisation of the practice by participants. In AI implementation in radiology, cognitive participation would involve enrolling radiologists, radiographers, and other staff into the new AI-enabled workflows, ensuring their active involvement and commitment to the changes. Collective action refers to the coordinated efforts of actors to enact the practice. It involves reshaping behaviours, employing objects, and reorganising relationships to achieve the practice's goals. In AI implementation, collective action would entail aligning the actions of various stakeholders to effectively utilise AI tools and technologies in radiological processes. Reflexive monitoring involves continuously evaluating the practice and its outcomes. It includes both formal and informal assessments by participants, focusing on normative elements and everyday understanding of the practice. In the context of AI implementation, reflexive monitoring would entail ongoing evaluation of the impact of AI on radiological processes, adjusting practices based on feedback, and ensuring continuous improvement. However, important to consider is that the NPT model assumes that the infrastructure and technology are arranged, as it focuses on the cognitive and behavioural aspects of groups and individuals with new technology. The NPT can provide department management with an improved understanding on technology adoption for the purpose of creating targeted change initiatives along with the implementation of new technology [34], such as AI.

2.3 Position of Radiology in the Hospital

2.3.1 The Role of the Radiology Department

Many of the changes set in motion by the digital revolution in radiology will be further driven with the active use of AI technology. In particular, the role of referring physicians in viewing digital images together with AI results will be enhanced. This means that referring physicians are also active stakeholders when implementing AI applications in clinical routine, as the role of clinical decision-making with AI also falls, at least in part, to them. Another significant aspect where AI applications can have an impact is full task automation, including automated reporting [35]. Through automation of tasks, workload can be significantly alleviated and radiologists can focus their expertise on more challenging cases and clinical decision-making. Some watch these developments with fear, thinking that automation will result in loss of control and reduced quality of radiological services, ultimately eliminating the need of a radiologist. Indeed, the first AI applications certified for autonomous use are already commercially available [36]. Although the use of AI will inevitably lead to the redistribution of tasks and professional roles, it will also introduce new responsibilities for the radiology department. For instance, in the case of automated reporting, the radiology department will be actively involved in designing such AI-enhanced workflows, ensuring that tasks delegated to other professions are performed with appropriate training, oversight, and quality assurance measures in place to maintain the highest standards of patient care and safety [22]. Furthermore, the department of radiology can coordinate communication and collaboration among members of the healthcare team, which are also essential for successful implementation and execution of such AI-enhanced workflows within the radiology department. It is important to note that the details regarding the implementation and the extent to which such automated reporting workflows can be used will differ across countries and depend on constraints dictated by local legislation.

2.3.2   Re-distributing Work

While AI technology can assist in alleviating workload for radiology staff, its optimal use also requires re-evaluation and potentially restructuring of work-related tasks in the radiological workflow [37]. As a consequence, professional roles and domains may undergo changes, leading to the redistribution of tasks among various professions. This shift can bring about financial benefits through delegating tasks to less costly personnel, while concurrently enhancing job satisfaction by providing professionals with new tasks and responsibilities. Within the radiology department, task-differentiation can be done by means of introducing new clinical and technological professions, such as the physician assistant and nurse practitioner, or by retraining existing professions, for example radiographers to perform specific image analysis and reporting tasks [38]. Indeed, an increase in non-physician practitioners (NPPs) has been observed over the years [39], contributing to improved patient care and productivity in radiology consult practice [40]. It is expected that the introduction of AI will further drive task-differentiation, where automation will play a key role in how work-related tasks will be assigned to different disciplines [38]. Important changes are already visible at the level of image acquisition, where several vendors of imaging equipment started to implement AI technology for the purpose of automating processes around image acquisition. Acquiring medical images is a highly specialist task in the radiological workflow that requires specific expertise from well-trained radiographers. With the support of AI technology that can automate patient positioning [41], optimal selection of image acquisition settings and scan range, many routine work-related tasks of radiographers could potentially be done by radiographer assistants, while radiographers can focus on more complex imaging protocols. In turn, with the support of AI technology, radiographers could focus more on complex image acquisition protocols and radiological tasks such as image processing and reporting, thereby reducing workload for radiologists.

2.4   Organisational Aspects of AI Implementation

The integration and operational deployment of AI requires careful orchestration of tasks across diverse disciplines. Institutions often struggle with the task of aligning their organisational structure with the acquisition, implementation, and utilisation of AI. Given that each AI application is essentially an independent software application, its implementation requires the same procedure as any other regular software application. This includes drafting of a comprehensive programme, covering software requirements and risk assessment, ethical considerations [42], as well as the management of contractual processes, including legal [43], financial, and privacy considerations [22]. It also involves the establishment of data processing agreements and data protection impact assessments, ensuring the effective management of security aspects [44]. With the implementation of multiple AI applications, coordinating efforts between project teams becomes essential. This coordination can be effectively executed by a dedicated innovation manager, tasked with coordinating and planning sessions involving clinicians, IT specialists, legal counsellors, security and privacy officers, and companies to steer the AI implementation process [22]. The innovation manager takes charge of assembling multidisciplinary project teams dedicated to designing AI-enhanced workflows. Within the project team, the innovation manager facilitates communication between various disciplines and regularly provides progress reports to department management. Through regular progress reporting, the department management can prioritise specific projects and allocate additional resources to expedite AI implementation in the event of delays or bottlenecks.

2.4.1 The Innovation Committee

While the innovation manager plays a crucial role in streamlining the acquisition and implementation process of AI applications, effective portfolio management requires broader consensus. Portfolio management can be delegated to a department-wide innovation committee, comprising departmental leadership (i.e., department head, medical and financial managers) and representatives from various disciplines and groups within the department. The innovation committee is responsible for prioritising submitted innovation projects based on their initial value propositions, as outlined in concise project proposals commonly referred to as 'one-pagers' or 'templated intake forms' [22].

The committee evaluates the submissions and approves projects aligning with the department's strategic plan. Upon approval, the innovation manager and project teams move forward with the execution of the endorsed projects, while the innovation committee has the authority to allocate resources strategically to enhance the success rate of the project. Furthermore, the innovation committee plays an active role in monitoring project progress and provides assistance in the event of significant delays, either by allocating additional resources or finding solutions to overcome obstacles.

While everyone within and outside the radiology department can submit innovation projects to the innovation committee, designated individuals (such as radiologists and radiographers) can be assigned to take the lead in scouting the market for available technology. These individuals, known as 'innovation champions,' play a crucial role in maintaining a steady flow of new ideas by motivating their peers. Moreover, they are instrumental in communicating new implementations to their colleagues and promoting the active adoption of emerging technology. In essence, they play a crucial role in persuading the early and late majority as well as laggards.

2.4.2 Institutional-Wide Organisation

To effectively scale the adoption of AI technology in healthcare, it is crucial to implement organisational changes beyond the radiology department. Establishing an institution-wide clinical AI implementation group serves as a centralised hub for coordinating efforts across diverse departments [22]. This group acts as a pivotal point for disseminating information and sharing knowledge in specific domains such as legal, privacy, technology, and security, derived from various AI use cases. This can be organised by including several lead experts from different relevant fields that bring specialised knowledge together for others to use in new innovations. By facilitating communication, providing training, and overseeing evaluation, the AI implementation group plays a strategic role in planning, governance, and change management efforts. By establishing a close collaboration with key departments and faculties, implementation of AI can be performed more effectively, safely, and responsible. This will ultimately create a culture of innovation and collaboration that contributes to improving patient care and outcomes through the holistic adoption of AI technology.

2.5 Conclusions

While AI presents significant opportunities for advancement in radiology, it also demands careful consideration of its impact on the workforce, patient care, and the broader healthcare ecosystem. Future efforts should focus on creating a culture of innovation and collaboration that embraces AI technology as a partner in clinical care. By doing so, radiology departments can not only improve operational efficiencies and patient outcomes but also lead the way in this transformation. The journey towards AI-enhanced radiology is complex and ongoing, requiring a commitment to continuous learning, adaptation, and integration of new technologies into the fabric of radiological practice.

References

1. Smith-Bindman R, et al. Trends in use of medical imaging in US health care systems and in Ontario, Canada, 2000–2016. JAMA. 2019;322:843–56.
2. Milano MT, Mahesh M, Mettler FA, Elee J, Vetter RJ. Patient radiation exposure: imaging during radiation oncology procedures: executive summary of NCRP report no. 184. J Am Coll Radiol. 2020;17:1176–82.
3. Mettler FA Jr, et al. Use of radiology in U.S. general short-term hospitals: 1980–1990. Radiology. 1993;189:377–80.
4. Martella M, Lenzi J, Gianino MM. Diagnostic technology: trends of use and availability in a 10-year period (2011–2020) among sixteen OECD countries. Healthcare (Basel). 2023;11:2078.
5. Borgstede JP. Radiology: commodity or specialty. Radiology. 2008;247:613–6.
6. Lemke HU. Short history of PACS (part II: Europe). Eur J Radiol. 2011;78:177–83.
7. Rosenkrantz AB, et al. Clinical utility of quantitative imaging. Acad Radiol. 2015;22:33–49.
8. Parikh JR, Bender CE. How radiology leaders can address burnout. J Am Coll Radiol. 2021;18:679–84.
9. Shanafelt TD, et al. Changes in burnout and satisfaction with work-life integration in physicians and the general US working population between 2011 and 2017. Mayo Clin Proc. 2019;94:1681–94.
10. Fawzy NA, et al. Incidence and factors associated with burnout in radiologists: A systematic review. Eur J Radiol Open. 2023;11:100530.
11. Singh N, et al. Occupational burnout among radiographers, sonographers and radiologists in Australia and New Zealand: Findings from a national survey. J Med Imaging Radiat Oncol. 2017;61:304–10.
12. Agrawal S, Conway PH. Aligning emergency care with the triple aim: opportunities and future directions after healthcare reform. Healthc Pap. 2014;2:184–9.
13. Bergevin Y, et al. Transforming regions into high-performing health systems toward the triple aim of better health, better care and better value for Canadians. Healthc Pap. 2016;16:34–52.

14. Obucina M, et al. The application of triple aim framework in the context of primary healthcare: a systematic literature review. Health Policy. 2018;122:900–7.
15. Berwick DM, Nolan TW, Whittington J. The triple aim: care, health, and cost. Health Aff. 2008;27:759–69.
16. Bodenheimer T, Sinsky C. From triple to quadruple aim: care of the patient requires care of the provider. Ann Fam Med. 2014;12:573–6.
17. Enzmann DR. Radiology's value chain. Radiology. 2012;263:243–52.
18. Dreyer KJ, Geis JR. When machines think: radiology's next frontier. Radiology. 2017;285:713–8.
19. Dzobo K, Adotey S, Thomford NE, Dzobo W. Integrating artificial and human intelligence: a partnership for responsible innovation in biomedical engineering and medicine. OMICS. 2020;24:247–63.
20. Hosny A, Parmar C, Quackenbush J, Schwartz LH, Aerts HJWL. Artificial intelligence in radiology. Nat Rev Cancer. 2018;18:500–10.
21. Montagnon E, et al. Deep learning workflow in radiology: a primer. Insights Imaging. 2020;11:22.
22. Kim B, Romeijn S, van Buchem M, Mehrizi MHR, Grootjans W. A holistic approach to implementing artificial intelligence in radiology. Insights Imaging. 2024;15:22.
23. Mehrizi MHR, et al. How do providers of artificial intelligence (AI) solutions propose and legitimize the values of their solutions for supporting diagnostic radiology workflow? A technography study in 2021. Eur Radiol. 2023;33:915–24.
24. Rezazade Mehrizi MH, van Ooijen P, Homan M. Applications of artificial intelligence (AI) in diagnostic radiology: a technography study. Eur Radiol. 2021;31:1805–11.
25. Parikh RB, Helmchen LA. Paying for artificial intelligence in medicine. NPJ Digit Med. 2022;5:63.
26. Brynjolfsson E, Rock D, Syverson C. The productivity J-curve: how intangibles complement general purpose technologies. Am Econ J Macroecon. 2021;13:333–72.
27. Babina T, Fedyk A, He A, Hodson J. Artificial intelligence, firm growth, and product innovation. J Financ Econ. 2024;151:103745. https://doi.org/10.1016/j.jfineco.2023.103745.
28. Mello-Thoms C, Mello CAB. Clinical applications of artificial intelligence in radiology. Br J Radiol. 2023;96:20221031.
29. Huisman M, et al. An international survey on AI in radiology in 1041 radiologists and radiology residents part 1: fear of replacement, knowledge, and attitude. Eur Radiol. 2021;31:7058–66.
30. Rogers EM. Diffusion of innovations. 5th ed. Simon and Schuster; 2003.
31. Benson T. Digital innovation evaluation: user perceptions of innovation readiness, digital confidence, innovation adoption, user experience and behaviour change. BMJ Health Care Inform. 2019;26

32. May C. Towards a general theory of implementation. Implement Sci. 2013;8:18.
33. May C, Finch T. Implementing, embedding, and integrating practices: an outline of normalization process theory. Sociology. 2009;43:535–54.
34. Davis S. Ready for prime time? Using normalization process theory to evaluate implementation success of personal health records designed for decision making. Front Digit Health. 2020;2:575951.
35. Monshi MMA, Poon J, Chung V. Deep learning in generating radiology reports: a survey. Artif Intell Med. 2020;106:101878.
36. Miró Catalina Q, Fuster-Casanovas A, Solé-Casals J, Vidal-Alaball J. Developing an artificial intelligence model for reading chest X-rays: protocol for a prospective validation study. JMIR Res Protoc. 2022;11:e39536.
37. Jha S. Algorithms at the gate-radiology's AI adoption dilemma. JAMA. 2023;330:1615–6.
38. Hardy M, Harvey H. Artificial intelligence in diagnostic imaging: impact on the radiography profession. Br J Radiol. 2020;93:20190840.
39. Santavicca S, Hughes DR, Rosenkrantz AB, Rubin E, Duszak R Jr. Radiology practices employing nurse practitioners and physician assistants: characteristics and trends from 2017 through 2019. J Am Coll Radiol. 2022;19:746–53.
40. Virarkar M, et al. PAs and NPs improve patient care and productivity in a radiology consult practice. JAAPA. 2022;35:46–51.
41. Manava P, et al. Optimized camera-based patient positioning in CT: impact on radiation exposure. Investig Radiol. 2023;58:126–30.
42. Geis JR, et al. Ethics of artificial intelligence in radiology: summary of the joint European and North American multisociety statement. Radiology. 2019;293:436–40.
43. Mezrich JL. Is artificial intelligence (AI) a pipe dream? Why legal issues present significant hurdles to AI autonomy. AJR Am J Roentgenol. 2022;219:152–6.
44. Kondylakis H, et al. Data infrastructures for AI in medical imaging: a report on the experiences of five EU projects. Eur Radiol Exp. 2023;7:20.

Planning and Goal Setting

3

Elmar Kotter

Key Points

- The demonstration of the need for change is not a mere convention; it is the crucial element on which the entire framework for the integration of AI will be based. This stage ensures consistency, direction, and purpose for radiology departments as they progress towards the adoption of AI technology.
- Goal setting is the foundation for integrating AI into radiology, providing direction, clarity, and a roadmap to ensure that concerted efforts bring about the desired change. By providing clarity, direction, and a roadmap, it ensures that efforts are systematic, concerted and deliver the desired transformation.
- A well-defined scope, based on extensive research and stakeholder consultation, provides a clear direction. This approach reduces uncertainty, sets realistic expectations,

E. Kotter (✉)
Department of Diagnostic and Interventional Radiology,
Medical Center—University of Freiburg,
Freiburg, Germany
e-mail: elmar.kotter@uniklinik-freiburg.de

© The Author(s), under exclusive license to Springer Nature Switzerland AG 2024
E. Ranschaert et al. (eds.), *AI Implementation in Radiology*, Imaging Informatics for Healthcare Professionals,
https://doi.org/10.1007/978-3-031-68942-0_3

and ensures that the process of integrating AI into radiology is focused, targeted, and productive.
- While AI offers transformative potential for radiology, it cannot be treated as a 'fire-and-forget' solution. To ensure sustainable, ethical, and effective adoption, AI requires robust governance structures, a proactive approach to addressing challenges, and a commitment to continuous learning and improvement.

3.1 Introduction

It is important to understand that introducing AI into radiology is not just about technological innovation. It is more fundamentally about managing and orchestrating the multitude of changes that this integration will cause. As Kotter's seminal work on change management shows, achieving sustainable change requires a clear vision, strategy, and meticulous planning [1]. It requires a departure from linear thinking and embracing a systems thinking approach where different components, from technology to people, interact in a coordinated symphony of change [2].

This chapter explores the many facets involved in planning and goal setting, as radiology departments worldwide grapple with the opportunities and challenges of AI. It looks at understanding the 'why' behind the change, setting clear goals, and methodically creating a roadmap to ensure the sustainable and beneficial integration of AI into radiology [3]. In outlining this path, the chapter aims to provide guidance for the transformational journey of AI implementation [4].

3.2 Establishing the Necessity for Change

Integrating AI into radiology requires a thorough understanding of the underlying reasons for doing so. It is not just about adopting cutting-edge technology; it is also about addressing inherent needs, solving persistent problems, and ultimately improving patient outcomes.

Historically, medical practice has been driven by the dual motivations of necessity and innovation [5]. In radiology, these motivations create a compelling context for discussing AI. Radiology departments have struggled with challenges such as increasing workloads, higher patient volumes, and the constant pursuit of diagnostic accuracy [6]. At the same time, it has become increasingly clear that traditional tools, no matter how sophisticated, have limitations. The capabilities of AI, which focus on pattern recognition, speed, and predictive analysis, can be advantageous compared to traditional radiology tools [7].

Additionally, the healthcare system is becoming more patient-centred and moving towards value-based care [8]. This shift means that healthcare organisations are measuring success based on comprehensive patient outcomes and experience (such as perceived quality of medical services, sense of being informed about decisions), rather than just procedural accuracy. As a result, the 'need for change' encompasses both the obstacles faced by radiology professionals and the demands of patients in a rapidly changing healthcare ecosystem.

One should keep in mind that there is a broader global context to this transformation. The digital changes that are transforming industries suggest that AI is not an option but rather a necessity to remain competitive and relevant [1, 9]. As a critical industry, healthcare cannot escape these market dynamics.

Recognising these needs is not enough. A methodical assessment of needs, which requires a thorough examination of existing competencies, drawbacks, and opportunities for progress, provides a secure foundation for the transition process [2]. This assessment ensures that AI is introduced based on explicit, workable requirements rather than on short-lived technological enchantment. By comparing the current state of radiology practices with the prospective benefits of AI (like reducing error rates in lung nodule detection or speeding up quantitative tasks), stakeholders will be able to establish a compelling rationale for change, one that is consistent with the goals of clinicians and the well-being of patients [3].

The demonstration of the need for change is not a mere convention; it is the crucial element on which the entire framework for the integration of AI will be based. This stage ensures consistency, direction, and purpose for radiology departments as they progress towards the adoption of AI technology [4].

3.3   Setting Clear Objectives

In the rapidly changing healthcare landscape, setting a clear direction is paramount. The integration of AI into radiology should not be undertaken lightly or impulsively. It requires careful planning that is supported by specific goals that are measurable and actionable [8].

According to Kotter's eight-step change management model, creating a sense of urgency, a guiding coalition, and a clear vision and strategy are critical steps [10]. Applying this principle to the integration of AI in radiology highlights the importance of setting focused goals.

The first point to consider is *specificity*. In the vast field of AI, which capabilities do we want to exploit? AI can serve different purposes in radiology, ranging from predictive analytics to automating mundane tasks and refining diagnostic accuracy [11]. It is therefore important to narrow the focus. Is the goal to streamline workflows or to develop new diagnostic methods? *Precise objectives* act as an anchor, ensuring that efforts do not drift aimlessly.

However, being precise without being *measurable* can lead to abstract goals. Objectives need to be linked to metrics, and metrics need to be linked to objectives [7]. For example, if the goal is to improve the speed of diagnosis, what is the target percentage increase? What is the expected impact on patient waiting times? Benchmarks provide accountability and a clear measure of success.

Achievability is what makes objectives realistic. Although it may be tempting to set ambitious goals, practical constraints related to technology, infrastructure, and human resources should be taken into account [12]. Learning from pilots, case studies or peer institutions can provide valuable insights into what is achievable in the immediate and long term.

Alignment is ensured through *relevance*. Goals should be harmoniously integrated with the broader goals of the radiology department and, by extension, the healthcare institution as a whole [4]. AI should not be pursued in isolation, but rather should complement and enhance the mission and vision of the department.

Introducing *urgency*, timeliness plays an important role. Radiology departments should establish a phased timeline, identifying milestones to track progress and maintain momentum [1].

Goal setting is the foundation for integrating AI into radiology, providing direction, clarity, and a roadmap to ensure that concerted efforts bring about the desired change. By providing clarity, direction and a roadmap, it ensures that efforts are systematic, concerted and deliver the desired transformation [3].

3.4   Defining the Scope of Changes

Defining the scope is like drawing a roadmap for a journey. It provides a clear view of the start and end points, the route to be taken and the milestones to be achieved [1]. In the context of integrating AI into radiology, this means having a comprehensive understanding of the range and extent of changes—technological, procedural, and human—that the department intends to make.

Defining the scope starts with understanding the range of applications for AI. Radiology, with its diverse sub-disciplines, offers many opportunities for AI. From neuroradiology to interventional radiology, AI has the potential to be used in a range of applications in radiology [7]. Is the department's goal a comprehensive overhaul, or is the focus more niche, targeting specific procedures or techniques? The scope will determine the extent of change.

Depth is the next aspect to consider. Once the scope has been identified, what is the depth of change, i.e. how profound are the changes for an activity that is within the scope of changes? For example, if AI is introduced to mammography, are the changes limited to assisting with image analysis, or do they extend to predictive analytics for patient tracking and follow-up [13]? Depth reveals the intricacies and multiple layers of change.

The time dimension includes the duration and phasing of the change. Rapid integration can bring quick benefits but can also be disruptive. A phased approach may take longer, but may allow for course correction and adaptability [4]. Radiology departments should conceptualise short- (1–3 years), medium- (2–5 years), and long-term (5–12 years) timelines for AI adoption, drawing insights from McKinsey's three horizons of growth [14]. This conceptualisation helps to manage the visions and guide conversation by showing the stakeholders the grand innovation plan.

Finally, the human aspect, arguably the most important factor, should also be considered. The scope must take into account the roles that may be affected, redefined, or made redundant. It is essential that the scope includes training, upskilling, and transition plans for staff to ensure that human resources are aligned with technological change [8].

A well-defined scope, based on extensive research and stakeholder consultation, provides a clear direction. This approach reduces uncertainty, sets realistic expectations, and ensures that the process of integrating AI into radiology is focused, targeted, and productive [3].

3.5   Determining the Desired Outcomes

Integrating AI into radiology is not just about using complex algorithms or demonstrating advanced technology; it is primarily about achieving tangible, beneficial outcomes that can revolutionise patient care and improve operational efficiency [8]. Collectively identifying and agreeing on these desired outcomes are therefore critical aspects of the AI adoption process, providing a clear vision of what a successful outcome would look like. For AI in radiology, one possible categorisation of outcomes could be:

1. **Clinical outcomes**: Radiology is fundamentally concerned with accurate medical diagnosis and patient welfare. The most important clinical outcomes would include
   - Improved diagnostic accuracy: Using AI to reduce the number of false positive and negative diagnoses, resulting in more accurate diagnoses [7].
   - Predictive analysis: AI can be used for early detection of potential medical problems based on imaging patterns, facilitating preventative care [13].
   - Treatment planning: AI can provide insights into the potential success of different treatment options based on imaging data [15].
2. **Operational outcomes**: Radiology departments, like any other organisational entity, strive for effectiveness and productivity. AI can play an important role in
   - Optimising workflow: Improving the efficiency of the radiology process by streamlining processes and reducing bottlenecks [16].
   - Resource allocation: This involves predicting peak times and resource requirements to enable better allocation of staff and equipment [4].
   - Cost efficiency: Automating routine tasks and reducing errors with AI can lead to significant cost savings [17].
3. **Experiential outcomes**: Despite the dominance of technology in this era, the personal connection remains invaluable. Intended outcomes in this area could include
   - Improved experience for radiologists: By reducing manual and repetitive tasks, radiologists can focus on more complex diagnostics and patient interactions [18].
   - Improved experience for patients: Faster diagnosis, more consistent communication, and better outcomes can significantly enrich the patient journey [19].

However, as Kotter emphasised in his framework, the achievement of results is an ongoing process; it requires regular check-ins, evaluations and improvements based on feedback and changing circumstances [1]. This iterative approach ensures that outcomes remain applicable, achievable, and aligned with the broader goals of the health care organisation.

Establishing desired outcomes provides a guiding principle for the AI integration process in radiology, ensuring that every effort, resource, and change are aligned with the desired success.

3.6   The Importance of Feedback

In any transformative journey, and especially in the integration of AI in radiology, feedback is critical for iterative improvement. It reflects ongoing efforts, provides insights, highlights blind spots, and suggests ways to improve [8].

The nature of AI is based on iterative learning, where models improve with more data and feedback [20]. Similarly, the successful integration of AI in radiology requires continuous input from various stakeholders.

Once feedback is collected, it needs to be systematically analysed and actionable insights derived. Implementing changes based on feedback ensures that the journey of AI integration is adaptive and responsive. It also fosters a culture of continuous learning and improvement, which is essential for the ever-evolving field of AI [21].

If feedback is actively sought, carefully analysed and strategically acted upon, it can guide the process of AI integration in radiology, ensuring that it remains aligned with both clinical excellence and user experience (Table 3.1).

Table 3.1 Types and mechanisms of feedback

Types of feedback		Feedback mechanisms	
Technical feedback	Refers to the performance of AI tools. Are the algorithms making accurate predictions? Is the system stable or are there technical issues? This type of feedback is essential for IT teams and AI vendors [22]	Regular reviews	Establishing regular reviews in which teams discuss the AI integration process can provide structured feedback. These sessions, guided by pre-set agendas, can become forums for cross-departmental dialogue [3]
Clinical feedback	Radiologists and other medical professionals provide insight into the clinical relevance of AI results. This feedback loop can be a valuable training resource to improve the AI system's algorithms [23]	Surveys	Anonymous surveys can encourage honest feedback, especially on sensitive issues or perceived difficulties. They can be tailored to different stakeholders, such as radiologists, support staff or patients [18]
Operational feedback	This feedback takes into account insights from administrative staff, as well as concerns about workflow integration, system interfaces, and overall daily utility [4]	Real-time reporting tools	The use of tools that provide immediate feedback, particularly on technical challenges, can speed up problem resolution [24]. Ideally, the feedback on AI results should be automated and integrated in the radiologists reading process
Patient feedback	Patients, the ultimate beneficiaries, can provide feedback on their experience, the clarity of reports, and perceived changes in the quality of care following AI integration [19]	Patient forums	Engaging patients through forums or focus groups can provide valuable insights from a user experience perspective [19]

3.7   User Experience

Beyond technical processes and clinical outcomes, the advent of AI in radiology has a profound impact on the user experience (UX). While the technical achievements of AI are undoubtedly transformative, if the end-user—radiologist, support staff, or patient—finds the system difficult to navigate or interpret, its true potential remains untapped [19].

In the context of integrating AI into radiology, UX refers to how different users interact with the AI system, the ease with which they interact, and their overall satisfaction. User interfaces should be clean, easy to understand, and use [21]. Users range from radiologists to technologists, administrators and patients [24].

A well-designed UX allows easy and efficient interaction with the AI systems, thus increasing operational efficiency [25]. Intuitive and well-designed systems can significantly reduce user errors, increasing the accuracy and reliability of results. A positive user experience can boost confidence in the AI system, creating a more welcoming environment for technological change [3]. Real-time feedback can make AI tools more engaging [26]. Customisation of the UX allows users to tailor and personalise their UX [27]. Involving end-users early in the planning and iterative testing ensures that the system becomes more user centred [23, 28]. Initial training and continuous support of users can ease the introduction of AI systems.

While the power of AI in radiology lies in its algorithms and predictions, its success in the real world is deeply intertwined with the user experience. A well-designed, user-centred approach can ensure that the integration of AI is smooth, effective, and welcomed by all.

3.8   Resource Allocation

Resource allocation is an essential component of any transformation project. Ensuring that adequate resources are allocated in a timely manner can have a significant impact on the success of AI integration in radiology. It is not just about financial resources, but also time, manpower, technical infrastructure, and ongoing training [8]. An overview on resource allocation is given in Table 3.2.

Table 3.2 Resource allocation

Types of resources	Allocation principles	Allocation challenges
Financial resources: The economic aspect is of crucial importance. This includes not only the cost of AI software and tools. It also includes potential infrastructure upgrades, training programmes, and ongoing maintenance costs [25]	*Prioritising:* Understand which stages or components of the integration process are most critical and allocate resources accordingly. This could mean prioritising initial training or ensuring a robust technical infrastructure is in place before the system goes live	*Limited resources:* Resources, especially funding, are often limited. Balancing needs while ensuring project success becomes critical [32]
Human resources: The involvement of different professionals—From radiologists and IT specialists to project managers and training coordinators—Is critical. Their roles, responsibilities, and time commitments need to be clearly defined [29]	*Flexibility:* AI integration is a dynamic process. It is important to maintain some flexibility in resource allocation to deal with unforeseen challenges or new requirements [10]	*Changing requirements:* As the integration process unfolds, some initial assumptions may change, leading to a reallocation of resources [33]
Technical infrastructure: Robust hardware, reliable software platforms, and a strong network infrastructure form the backbone of any AI integration process [17]	*Stakeholder involvement:* Involve key stakeholders in resource allocation decisions. Their insights can provide a more holistic view of what's needed and when [31]	*Stakeholder conflicts:* Different stakeholders may have different views on resource allocation, leading to potential conflict. Effective communication and a clear vision can help in such scenarios [22]
Time: Time is a nuanced resource. While it is important to maintain momentum, sufficient time must be allocated for stages such as testing, feedback, and refinement [3]	*Continuous monitoring:* Regularly assess whether resources are being used efficiently. Tools and methods such as the critical path method (CPM) or the programme evaluation and review technique (PERT) can be useful [1]	
Training materials: These can range from user manuals, online tutorials, workshops, or even external courses for in-depth knowledge [30]		

Integrating AI into radiology requires a comprehensive under-standing of the various resources involved. Each phase, from planning to implementation and monitoring, requires specific resources. Efficient resource allocation will ensure that the project runs smoothly, mitigate potential bottlenecks, and ensure that the system delivers optimal value [4].

Strategic resource allocation is not just about distributing resources, but optimising them to achieve the desired outcomes in the integration of AI in radiology. It's about using available resources to create a system that is effective, efficient, and sustainable.

3.9   Potential Risks

Inevitably, there are potential risks associated with any significant technological change, such as the integration of AI in radiology (Table 3.3). Recognising these risks, understanding their implica-

Table 3.3 Possible risks in integration AI technology in radiology

Technical complications, for instance, malfunctions in software or hardware incompatibility [34]
Human errors resulting from inadequate training or supervision
Organisational challenges such as resistance to change or insufficient communication channels
External factors such as regulatory changes or complications relating to vendors [35]
Resistance to adoption: Despite the potential benefits, clinicians may be reluctant to use AI tools, citing concerns about their reliability or the loss of human touch in diagnostics [22]
Incorrect diagnosis: AI models can pose direct risks to patients if they are not accurately trained, which may result in the misinterpretation of medical images [36]
Regulatory and ethical challenges: As AI is a relatively new phenomenon in healthcare, navigating the regulatory waters can be challenging
Concerns regarding data privacy: The need to ensure data privacy and security becomes paramount due to the extensive amount of data required by AI models [37]
Potential budget overruns: Budgets can be strained by unanticipated costs, prolonged integrations, or technology switches [29]
Operational disruptions: Poorly planned implementations can disrupt daily radiology operations, resulting in delays in patient care [38]

Table 3.4 Risk mitigation strategies

Risk mitigation strategies when implementing AI in radiology
Comprehensive planning: When all stakeholders provide inputs for detailed planning, it can forestall many potential risks [41]
Continuing education: Regular training sessions guarantee that users remain updated and minimise errors caused by human factors [42]
Thorough testing: Prior to complete implementation, AI models should undergo rigorous testing on diverse datasets to reduce misdiagnosis risks [19]
Transparent communication: Frequent updates regarding the integration process, its benefits, and addressing concerns can lower the opposition towards adoption [43]
Involving regulatory experts: As healthcare regulations regarding AI evolve with time, involving experts can instil compliance and predict the changes that lie ahead [44]

tions, and planning accordingly are essential for both the safety and success of implementation [8].

Establishing a structured approach to risk management that goes through identification, mitigation, and regular monitoring can effectively minimise potential risks. Frameworks such as PRINCE2 [39] or PMBOK [40] provide structured methodologies for managing risks in projects that involve AI integrations.

Although risks associated with AI integration in radiology are expected, they can still be mitigated (Table 3.4). By employing foresight, planning, and a commitment to continuous learning and adaptation, AI risks can be managed, thus guaranteeing the realisation of AI benefits without compromising the safety, ethics, or operational excellence.

3.10 Governance of AI in Radiology

Governance refers to the framework of rules, practices, and processes for directing and controlling AI systems in radiology. Effective governance ensures that AI operates reliably, ethically, and beneficially, balancing innovation with accountability [45]. Effective and responsible usage of AI in the radiology department heavily relies on its governance. Establishment of protocols, guidelines, and structures that oversee AI's lifecycle, from its introduction to continuous monitoring, and future possible evolutions, is essential for proper governance [19].

3.10.1 Essential Elements of AI Governance in Radiology

- Development of policies and protocols: Drafting transparent guidelines regarding AI's usage, the types of data it can process and its interplay with clinical decisions is vital. This should also consider ethical issues, particularly regarding patient data [46].
- Structures of oversight and accountability: Appointing dedicated committees or teams to supervise AI's performance, ensuring compliance to established protocols and making any necessary changes [47].
- Continuous monitoring and maintenance: Unlike traditional tools, AI learns and evolves. Regularly reviewing its decisions, updating its algorithms and ensuring it remain reliable are an essential task [48].
- Stakeholder engagement: Ensuring all stakeholders, from radiologists to patients, understands the role of AI and has channels to voice concerns or feedback is a crucial part of governance [49].
- Regulatory compliance: As healthcare AI regulations change, it is essential to ensure that AI systems comply with those regulations [50].

3.10.2 The Importance of Leadership in the Governance of AI

Good governance starts with leadership. Governance should be a priority for leadership. They must allocate required resources, emphasise its significance, and foster a culture of accountability. Their commitment establishes the overall tone for the department [51].

Challenges in AI Governance:

- The dynamic nature of AI: As AI continues to evolve, maintaining its adherence to set protocols can be challenging [52].
- Regulations that are continually evolving: As governments and institutions are grappling with the implications of AI, regulations may change, demanding the department to be more agile [53].
- Finding a balance between innovation and control: Overly stringent governance may curb innovation, whereas a far too relaxed approach could raise risks [54].
- Ensuring involvement of all relevant parties: As AI is a highly technical field, ensuring that all relevant parties truly understand and participate in its governance can be challenging [19].

While AI offers transformative potential for radiology, it cannot be treated as a 'fire-and-forget' solution. To ensure sustainable, ethical, and effective adoption, AI requires robust governance structures, a proactive approach to addressing challenges, and a commitment to continuous learning and improvement.

References

1. Kotter JP. Leading change. Harvard Business Press; 2012.
2. Senge PM. The fifth discipline: the art and practice of the learning organization. Currency; 2006.
3. Langlotz CP. Will artificial intelligence replace radiologists? Radiology. 2019;1(3):e190058.
4. Davenport TH, Ronanki R. Artificial intelligence for the real world. Harv Bus Rev. 2018;96(1):108–16.
5. Mazurowski MA. Artificial intelligence may cause a significant disruption to the radiology workforce. J Am Coll Radiol. 2019;16(8):1077–82.
6. Rubin GD. Artificial intelligence in medical imaging: harnessing a revolution. Radiology. 2019;293(2):277–8.
7. Hosny A, Parmar C, Quackenbush J, Schwartz LH, Aerts HJ. Artificial intelligence in radiology. Nat Rev Cancer. 2018;18(8):500–10.
8. Thrall JH, Li X, Li Q, Cruz C, Do S, Dreyer K, Brink J. Artificial intelligence and machine learning in radiology: opportunities, challenges, pitfalls, and criteria for success. J Am Coll Radiol. 2018;15(3):504–8.
9. Schwab K. The fourth industrial revolution. Currency; 2017.

10. Topol EJ. High-performance medicine: the convergence of human and artificial intelligence. Nat Med. 2019;25(1):44–56.

11. McDonald RJ, Schwartz KM, Eckel LJ, Diehn FE, Hunt CH, Bartholmai BJ, et al. The effects of changes in utilization and technological advancements of cross-sectional imaging on radiologist workload. Acad Radiol. 2015;22(9):1191–8.

12. Porter ME, Teisberg EO. Redefining health care: creating value-based competition on results. Harvard Business Press; 2006.

13. Yala A, Lehman C, Schuster T, Portnoi T, Barzilay R. A deep learning mammography-based model for improved breast cancer risk prediction. Radiology. 2019;292(1):60–6.

14. Baghai M, Coley S, White D. The alchemy of growth: practical insights for building the enduring enterprise. Perseus Books; 1999.

15. Bi WL, Hosny A, Schabath MB, Giger ML, Birkbak NJ, Mehrtash A, et al. Artificial intelligence in cancer imaging: clinical challenges and applications. CA Cancer J Clin. 2019;69(2):127–57.

16. Lee CS, Nagy PG. Cognitive and system factors contributing to diagnostic errors in radiology. AJR. 2013;201(3):611–7.

17. Lakhani P, Sundaram B. Deep learning at chest radiography: automated classification of pulmonary tuberculosis by using convolutional neural networks. Radiology. 2017;284(2):574–82.

18. European Society of Radiology (ESR). Impact of artificial intelligence on radiology: a EuroAIM survey among members of the European Society of Radiology. Insights Imaging. 2019;10(1):105.

19. Geis JR, Brady AP, Wu CC, Spencer J, Ranschaert E, Jaremko JL, et al. Ethics of artificial intelligence in radiology: summary of the joint European and North American multisociety statement. Insights Imaging. 2019;10(1):1–8.

20. LeCun Y, Bengio Y, Hinton G. Deep learning. Nature. 2015;521(7553):436–44.

21. Zaharchuk G, Gong E, Wintermark M, Rubin D, Langlotz CP. Deep learning in neuroradiology. Am J Neuroradiol. 2018;39(10):1776–84.

22. Kelly CJ, Karthikesalingam A, Suleyman M, Corrado G, King D. Key challenges for delivering clinical impact with artificial intelligence. BMC Med. 2019;17(1):1–9.

23. Wang S, Summers RM. Machine learning and radiology. Med Image Anal. 2012;16(5):933–51.

24. Jha S, Topol EJ. Adapting to artificial intelligence: radiologists and pathologists as information specialists. JAMA. 2016;316(22):2353–4.

25. Kohli M, Prevedello LM, Filice RW, Geis JR. Implementing machine learning in radiology practice and research. Am J Roentgenol. 2017;208(4):754–60.

26. Lee D, Yoon SN. Application of artificial intelligence-based technologies in the healthcare industry: opportunities and challenges. Int J Environ Res Public Health. 2021;18(1):271.

27. Sit C, Srinivasan R, Amlani A, Muthuswamy K, Azam A, Monzon L, Poon DS. Attitudes and perceptions of UK medical students towards artificial intelligence and radiology: a multicentre survey. Insights Imaging. 2020;11(1):1–6.
28. National Science and Technology Council (2016) Preparing for the future of artificial intelligence. White House Report https://obamawhitehouse. archives.gov/sites/default/files/whitehouse_files/microsites/ostp/NSTC/ preparing_for_the_future_of_ai.pdf. Accessed 31 Jan 2024
29. Kruskal JB, Berkowitz S, Geis JR, Kim W, Nagy P, Dreyer K. Big data and machine learning—strategies for driving this bus: a summary of the 2016 intersociety summer conference. J Am Coll Radiol. 2017;14(6):811–7.
30. Tang A, Tam R, Cadrin-Chênevert A, Guest W, Chong J, Barfett J, et al. Canadian Association of Radiologists white paper on artificial intelligence in radiology. Can Assoc Radiol J. 2018;69(2):120–35.
31. Prevedello LM, Erdal BS, Ryu JL, Little KJ, Demirer M, Qian S, White RD. Automated critical test findings identification and online notification system using artificial intelligence in imaging. Radiology. 2017;285(3):923–31.
32. Collado-Mesa F, Alvarez E, Arheart K. The role of artificial intelligence in diagnostic radiology: a survey at a single radiology residency training program. J Am Coll Radiol. 2018;15(12):1753–7.
33. Liew C. The future of radiology augmented with artificial intelligence: a strategy for success. Eur J Radiol. 2018;102:152–6.
34. Choy G, Khalilzadeh O, Michalski M, Do S, Samir AE, Pianykh OS, et al. Current applications and future impact of machine learning in radiology. Radiology. 2018;288(2):318–28.
35. van Leeuwen KG, Schalekamp S, Rutten MJ, van Ginneken B, de Rooij M. Artificial intelligence in radiology: 100 commercially available products and their scientific evidence. Eur Radiol. 2021;31(6):3797–804.
36. Park SH, Han K. Methodologic guide for evaluating clinical performance and effect of artificial intelligence technology for medical diagnosis and prediction. Radiology. 2018;286(3):800–9.
37. Hricak H. 2016 new horizons lecture: beyond imaging—radiology of tomorrow. Radiology. 2018;286(3):764–75.
38. Davenport T, Kalakota R. The potential for artificial intelligence in healthcare. Future Healthc J. 2019;6(2):94.
39. https://www.prince2.com/. Accessed 21 Apr 2024
40. https://www.pmi.org/pmbok-guide-standards/foundational/pmbok. Accessed 21 Apr 2024
41. Aerts HJ. Data science in radiology: a path forward. Clin Cancer Res. 2018;24(3):532–4.
42. Tajmir SH, Alkasab TK. Toward augmented radiologists: changes in radiology education in the era of machine learning and artificial intelligence. Acad Radiol. 2018;25(6):747–50.

43. Curtis C, Liu C, Bollerman TJ, Pianykh OS. Machine learning for predicting patient wait times and appointment delays. J Am Coll Radiol. 2018;15(9):1310–6.
44. Price WN II, Cohen IG. Privacy in the age of medical big data. Nat Med. 2019;25(1):37–43.
45. Larson DB, Magnus DC, Lungren MP, Shah NH, Langlotz CP. Ethics of using and sharing clinical imaging data for artificial intelligence: a proposed framework. Radiology. 2020;295(3):675–82.
46. Vayena E, Blasimme A, Cohen IG. Machine learning in medicine: addressing ethical challenges. PLoS Med. 2018;15(11):e1002689.
47. Char DS, Shah NH, Magnus D. Implementing machine learning in health care—addressing ethical challenges. N Engl J Med. 2018;378(11):981–3.
48. Mittelstadt B. Principles alone cannot guarantee ethical AI. Nat Mach Intell. 2019;1(11):501–7.
49. Reddy S, Allan S, Coghlan S, Cooper P. A governance model for the application of AI in health care. J Am Med Inform Assoc. 2020;27(3):491–7.
50. He J, Baxter SL, Xu J, Xu J, Zhou X, Zhang K. The practical implementation of artificial intelligence technologies in medicine. Nat Med. 2019;25(1):30–6.
51. Recht M, Dewey M, Dreyer K, Langlotz C, Niessen W, Prainsack B, Smith JJ. Integrating artificial intelligence into the clinical practice of radiology: challenges and recommendations. Eur Radiol. 2020;30(6):3576–84.
52. Pesapane F, Volonté C, Codari M, Sardanelli F. Artificial intelligence as a medical device in radiology: ethical and regulatory issues in Europe and the United States. Insights Imaging. 2018;9(5):745–53.
53. Gerke S, Minssen T, Cohen G. Ethical and legal challenges of artificial intelligence-driven healthcare. Artificial Intelligence in healthcare; 2020. p. 295–336.
54. Floridi L, Cowls J, Beltrametti M, Chatila R, Chazerand P, Dignum V, et al. AI4People—an ethical framework for a good AI society: opportunities, risks, principles, and recommendations. Mind Mach. 2018;28(4):689–707.

Stakeholder Engagement and Communication

4

Kayla Berigan, Tessa S. Cook ⓘ, and Erik Ranschaert ⓘ

> **Key Points**
> - **Governance** should include members from inside and outside of the radiology department who represent clinical and non-clinical personas.
> - **Interdisciplinary collaboration** should be fostered, which requires radiologists to be more visible within their organizations.

K. Berigan (✉)
University of Wisconsin School of Medicine and Public Health, Madison, WI, USA
e-mail: Kberigan@wisc.edu

T. S. Cook
Hospital of the University of Pennsylvania, Philadelphia, PA, USA
e-mail: Tessa.Cook@pennmedicine.upenn.edu

E. Ranschaert
Department of Radiology, St. Nikolaus Hospital, Eupen, Belgium

Faculty of Medicine and Health Sciences, Ghent University, Ghent, Belgium
e-mail: erik.ranschaert@ugent.be

© The Author(s), under exclusive license to Springer Nature Switzerland AG 2024
E. Ranschaert et al. (eds.), *AI Implementation in Radiology*, Imaging Informatics for Healthcare Professionals,
https://doi.org/10.1007/978-3-031-68942-0_4

- **Communication** should be bidirectional, clear, and multifaceted to strengthen relationships and build acceptance of change.
- **Education** is required for stakeholders from multiple personas. There are ample existing educational tools, but organizations can also develop their own content.

4.1   Introduction

Shortly after the dawn of the field of radiology in the early 1900s, the perceived identity of radiologists was threatened in the United States, as some fear it is now by the emergence of AI. Modern speculations of radiologists' imminent extinction, such as Geoffrey Hinton's 2016 depiction of them as the cartoon coyote who has unknowingly run off the cliff, have similarly inspired fear in the radiology community and perhaps cast doubt among the public about the value of radiologists.

Ironically, to combat this worrisome view of the future, the present-day radiology community must adopt a strategy that is the exact opposite of what was employed in the US at the turn of the twentieth century. Finding that they were perceived by the public and the medical community as tradespeople rather than medical professionals, American radiologists of the early 1900s abandoned the practice of acquiring images themselves and providing films directly to patients [1]. Indeed, the current practice of conveying imaging results to referring providers originated from a 1916 recommendation by the American Roentgen Ray Society, which hoped it would establish the role of the radiologist as a medical consultant [1].

The unfortunate consequences of this shift in practice are the isolation and invisibility of radiologists [1], not only to patients but to referring providers and other stakeholders on whom our field depends. In an era in which patients are more informed, pressures to improve outcomes while reducing costs are greater than ever, and medicine is becoming increasingly sub-specialized, the deconstruction of this isolated mindset has never been more crucial. Add to this the emergence of AI, and with it our growing reliance on industry partners and information services professionals, and the urgency for change only grows.

Implementing AI in a way that maximizes value to the provision of imaging services and does so within the broader context of healthcare delivery will require the radiology community to become expert at engaging a growing number of stakeholders. In contrast to the way some of the pioneers of our field retracted from visibility and engagement, the members of today's imaging team need to step out of the dark. While some would see this as a strategy for radiologists to defend their identity and irreplaceability *despite* the existence of AI, the authors present it as precisely what will *empower* radiologists to be leaders in AI's implementation. Rather than stop training radiologists, as Hinton recommended, we should stop training radiologists who exist in a silo.

Discussed herein are the various stakeholders involved in the successful implementation of AI, the establishment of a governance structure, and strategies for communication and education around AI adoption.

4.2 Developing a Governance Structure

John Kotter, a pioneer of change management theory in business, suggests that the second step in an effective change effort, is "creating a guiding coalition," which follows the initial step of "establishing a sense of urgency" (described as "Identification of the Need for Change" in Chap. 2) [2]. When it comes to AI implementation in healthcare, the guiding coalition often takes the form of an AI steering committee, which may also be called a governance group or innovation committee, as it is referred to in Chap. 2. Many hospitals will develop a hospital-wide AI steering committee with a vision and strategy meant to align the entire organization. Radiology departments may or may not choose to form their own AI steering committees in addition to participating in the hospital-wide committee [3]. In either case, it is critical that radiology leaders share a close working relationship with those from other departments, and even a separate radiology AI steering committee will often include members from other departments.

In selecting which stakeholders to include in the governance group, it is important to have four core attributes represented: clinical domain expertise, non-clinical domain expertise, proven leadership skills, and influence within the enterprise [2]. As shown in Fig. 4.1, the committee should be composed of individuals of various roles who bring one or more of these attributes to the group. Depending on whether the governance structure consists of a hospital-wide group with or without a separate radiology department committee, membership may include the hospital Chief Medical Information Officer (CMIO), Radiology Department Chair or Group President, referring provider department leaders, data scientists, IT director, IT analysts, a PACS manager, a radiology technologist leader, and a medical physicist. It is also advantageous to include a project manager who can assist with coordination and communication [4]. Lastly, while they may not consistently serve on the committee, members of the hospital legal, contracting, and ethics departments should be consulted periodically [4].

In addition to these leaders, it is important that the committee includes at least one local champion who understands firsthand the potential impact of various AI solutions, can speak to their integration into the workflow, and is motivated to drive change [5]. Local champions for the radiology department are typically radiologists with a specific interest in AI who can inspire and guide others toward adoption. Specifically, this may involve providing educational materials and creating opportunities for radiologists to interact with AI via test versions or demonstrations [5]. In so doing, local champions help to familiarize their colleagues with the use of AI tools and lower the threshold for others to join in the change effort [5]. As described below, local or clinical champions may play a central role in overseeing specific AI projects if the committee is tasked with many requests at once [4]. A greater number of individuals can become involved by including "rotating members" in the steering committee. This offers the dual benefit of fresh perspective and inclusion of those who feel reluctant to commit to permanent involvement but would be willing to make a temporary contribution.

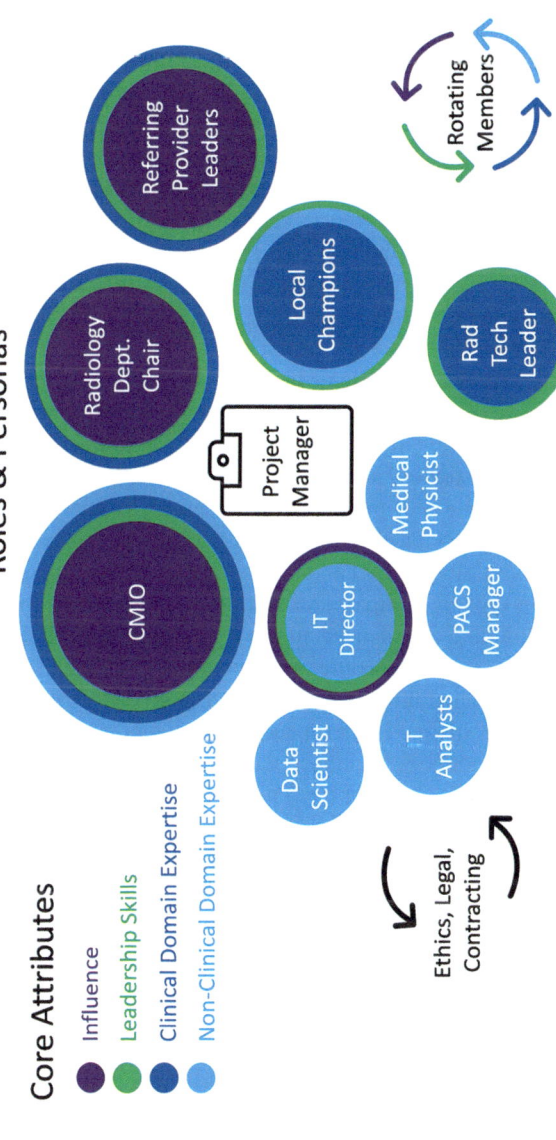

Fig. 4.1 Composition of an AI governance group. The group includes individuals responsible for planning, motivating team members, communicating within and across the group, and managing the project

After establishing the makeup of the AI governance group, it is essential to define the responsibilities of the group throughout the change process as a whole and the lifecycle of individual AI solutions. The first responsibility of the steering committee is to author clear vision and mission statements for AI adoption that resonate with the mission of the broader organization. The group should next develop a strategic plan which outlines how the vision and mission will be approached within a defined time period, such as 3–5 years, after which the plan should be updated given the rapid pace of advancement in the field [4]. The plan should include the articulation of specific goals as well as metrics by which progress on the goals can be assessed [4].

While the specific strategy of the committee will vary from institution to institution, their responsibilities will almost always include oversight of the selection process for which models to implement, allocation of needed resources for evaluation and deployment, oversight of the demonstration of return on investment, and facilitation of ongoing performance monitoring [3, 4, 6]. It is to be expected that the committee will be approached regarding a multitude of AI tools that various stakeholders are interested in implementing and/or testing at their institution. As such, the committee will need to have a defined prioritization strategy and selection procedure. This should be based on the submission of templated intake forms for each potential AI use case that describe pre-defined criteria such as business case, motivation, available model performance data, required model training and assessment data, and requested resources (technological, personnel, and financial) [4]. If the steering committee receives a large number of requests for model implementation, it may be necessary to form "project teams," for each request, composed of a subgroup of the larger committee, a clinical champion, and a member of the model development team (whether in-house or vendor-based) [4].

4.3   Defining Stakeholder Roles

Apart from the above members of an AI governance group, there are multiple additional stakeholders internal and external to the organization who need to be engaged. Both clinical and non-clinical personas should be represented, including radiologists, referring providers, patients, IT personnel, radiology technologists, purchasing teams, government authorities, and insurance companies.

4.3.1   Radiologists

Besides potentially acting as local champions and/or serving on an AI governance committee, there are multiple ways radiologists can contribute to the implementation of AI. In general, the greatest asset radiologists contribute is their familiarity and connection with the clinical domain. As such, they will be best positioned to coordinate the implementation of AI applications, including selection, evaluation, and post-deployment monitoring. Monitoring will include the practice of gatekeeping, likely integrated into daily workflow, which is discussed in more detail later in the chapter [5, 6]. These types of engagement which will be common to most radiologists as AI becomes broadly implemented will not necessarily require a high level of technical AI expertise. Rather, it will be essential for radiologists to be familiar with basic AI principles, analogous to their need to understand the fundamentals of medical physics in order to interpret images, troubleshoot issues with image quality, and conduct imaging research [7].

Some radiologists may choose to become more engaged in the development of new AI applications, often by partnering with engineers, developers, and data scientists. Others may become involved in AI business ventures, in which case their role could take a variety of forms, such as scientific collaborator, medical advisor, inventor, startup company founder, or vendor employee [8].

4.3.2   Referring Clinicians

Like radiologists, referring providers offer clinical expertise that is critical to the implementation of AI. Their knowledge of the impact of AI models on clinical decision-making and their direct exposure to patient outcomes make them well-suited to ensure AI solutions serve their intended purposes. In some cases, referring providers will have more established working relationships with hospital leadership, making them better-positioned to advocate for the value of AI. The counter to this, which the radiology community should look to avoid, is that in some cases referring providers may advocate for the implementation of imaging AI tools directly to hospital leadership without radiologist input [3]. These tools could be inserted into radiologists' workflow without their prior knowledge, or worse, be designed to bypass radiologists altogether. In either case, the result could be highly unfavorable. This underscores the importance of cultivating a collaborative relationship with referring providers and adopting an interdisciplinary, hospital-wide AI implementation vision and governance structure from day one.

An additional advantage of including referring providers in the AI change effort is that, for the most part, they have more direct interaction with patients. As such, if referring providers are informed and supportive of AI adoption, they can facilitate patient trust and acceptance of AI's role in their care. This should include offering opportunities for patients to learn about AI, ask questions, and voice concerns. Forums for this to take place, in addition to clinical encounters, could include patient focus groups, patient experience surveys, and print or electronic educational content. It is to be expected that patients will need this support, as prior research has shown that patients have reservations about AI making care decisions, particularly if unassisted by a provider [9–12]. In one study conducted by the Pew Research Center in 2022, the percentage of patients expressing discomfort with AI playing a role in their healthcare was greatest in patients with little or no familiarity with AI [12]. This highlights the important role that patient education can play in increasing acceptance of AI.

4.3.3   Patients

Specific patient concerns that have been cited in the literature include data privacy, the risk of discrimination due to algorithm bias, loss of human connection with providers, and liability for adverse outcomes [11, 12]. Transparency and open communication are essential if the medical community is to maintain a trusting relationship with patients as AI becomes an integral part of patient care. This is true not only when it comes to patients directly experiencing AI in their own care but also the use of deidentified patient data for model development. While patients have generally expressed approval of the use of deidentified data to serve the common good, they have also emphasized a desire that data sharing be voluntary, transparent, and open to patient input as to which data is shared and with whom. It has been suggested that AI disclosure guidelines are developed and that healthcare organizations are prepared to discuss the disclosure of deidentified data with patients [11].

4.3.4   Radiology Technologists (Radiographers)

Another group within the clinical team that will be impacted by the implementation of AI is radiology technologists (radiographers). Already, tools are emerging which will be integrated into technologists' workflow, such as those that aim to improve image quality, acquisition protocols, patient positioning, recognition of equipment malfunction, or image post-processing [13, 14]. Implementing these will require training technologists on their operation and monitoring [13, 14]. While training on fundamental AI principles will likely become increasingly incorporated into technologist training and certification programs, education for existing technologists will also need to be provided, potentially by radiology departments, national societies, and industry [14].

Like it does for radiologists, AI presents an opportunity for the role of technologists to evolve rather than being replaced. As this occurs, technologists should be empowered as integral members of the team and the change effort. The creation of a new role has even been suggested, the "AI Technologist," who would regularly test models and provide quality assurance on their outputs [15]. This model would be analogous to the way technologists already test equipment against performance standards, for example, in mammography and nuclear medicine. Technologist staffing will also be impacted as the use of AI increases. As some components of image acquisition become automated and efficiencies gained from AI result in increased patient throughput, technologists may be more likely to be required to function across multiple modalities in order to balance staffing with the changing workload [13].

4.3.5 Medical Physicists

AI is being applied to multiple components of the domain of medical physicists, including optimization of image quality, dose calibration, quantitative imaging, and radiotherapy treatment planning [16–18]. As such, the expertise of medical physicists will be crucial to AI implementation efforts. In many cases, this will involve applying their existing functions of modality and image quality control to the AI models that support related functions. Furthermore, because the performance and generalizability of machine learning models are often sensitive to changes in acquisition protocols, medical physicists will be instrumental in identifying and mitigating the effects of inconsistencies in technical image parameters on model performance [16]. Lastly, because their role has always been to work with an interdisciplinary team to ensure safe and consistent performance of technological tools, medical physicists are naturally positioned to assume the same role among stakeholders involved in AI implementation. To meet these evolving demands of the field, task groups and educational curricula have been developed by European medical physics societies, for example, the European Federation of Organizations for Medical Physics (EFOMP) working group on AI in Medical Physics and the Italian Association of Medical Physics (AIFM) AI for Medical Physics (AI4MP) group [16–18].

4.3.6 Hospital IT Professionals

PACS managers and other hospital IT professionals will clearly also experience changes in the amount and type of work demanded of them as AI implementation takes place. The degree to which this requires upskilling of existing employees, recruiting new individuals with AI expertise, or a combination thereof, will depend on the scale and nature of the organization's AI strategy. Organizations that aim to primarily implement purchased solutions with significant vendor support for installation and performance monitoring may not require dedicated radiology software developers, unlike those who wish to build AI in-house [6]. In-house developers, along with PACS administrators and possibly medical physicists, can also be useful when it comes to overseeing model performance in departments that have implemented multiple models and wish to track performance data using an AI dashboard. Considerations regarding an AI dashboard that will need to be determined, likely with input from the governance committee, include: what data is made available, how it is presented, and by whom it is maintained.

4.3.7 Other Stakeholders

Regardless of any given department's level of in-house IT staffing, vendors (or members of the model development team, for in-house applications) should be prepared to support every phase of their products' implementation and ongoing monitoring [6]. Members of the AI governance committee may find themselves needing to articulate these and other critical components of the value proposition to members of the purchasing team (hospital Chief Information Officer, Procurement Team), who may not have a high degree of familiarity with imaging-related AI [19].

The cost of AI products and the accompanying services are multifactorial and depend heavily on negotiation. Various contractual and pricing models exist (discussed in more detail in Chaps. 5 and 8) with different options for the exchange of value between the parties involved. For example, academic institutions may engage in collaborative research arrangements with vendors, or pharmaceutical companies producing AI widgets may offer them in exchange for purchase of other products, such as contrast agents. It is important to consider the ethical issues of patient privacy and data sharing when engaging in these arrangements. This will require engaging hospital ethics, compliance, and IRB personnel as discussed in detail in Chap. 6 [3].

When considering the return on investment of AI applications, additional groups to engage are government authorities and insurance companies, as they will dictate reimbursement and the regulatory environment [20]. Both may be willing to support the cost of AI implementation and utilization, if felt to offer sufficient value to justify the cost, such as by improving population health or patient outcomes. This will require institutions to generate data demonstrating said value and advocate to payers and government authorities. One example of collaboration among these stakeholders is the Netherlands' "Artificial Intelligence for Imaging (AIFI)" initiative. This project brings together Dutch insurance companies, the Radiological Society of the Netherlands (NVvR), 5 Dutch hospital pilot sites, and VZVZ, an organization responsible for the development and management of data exchange in healthcare. The goal of AIFI is to test the feasibility of a national radiology AI infrastructure supporting the evaluation of AI products with respect to clinical impact, technical requirements, and cost-benefit analyses of various purchasing models [21].

Considering all of the above stakeholders that are involved in undertaking the adoption of AI, it goes without saying that structural adaptations will need to be made within the enterprise. Even before pursuing the implementation of specific AI applications, it is crucial for the governance committee to spend significant time and effort considering what is needed by way of training existing staff, recruiting personnel to fill new roles, and strengthening relationships with groups inside and outside of the organization. Doing so will require highly effective communication and education strategies, discussed in the remainder of this chapter.

4.4   Communication Strategies

As alluded to in the above discussion on stakeholder roles and in the following section on education strategies, change leadership calls for a communication strategy that is bidirectional and transparent. The importance of this is emphasized in John Kotter's discussion of the sixth step in his change management model, "Communicating the Change Vision [2]." Open communication channels, Kotter argues, encourage honest dialogue about the challenges and opportunities facing the organization, thereby increasing trust and mutual understanding.

Effective communication in the change process can make or break the translation of the vision into action. As Kotter points out, the communication of a change vision is what creates "a shared sense of a desirable future," thereby "gaining understanding and commitment to a new direction." Among the challenges involved in doing so, are letting go of the status quo, willingness to make short-term sacrifices for long-term gains, and competing for the attention of employees who already receive an enormous volume of communication as part of routine operations.

Fortunately, Kotter offers seven pieces of practical advice to combat these challenges, depicted in Fig. 4.2: simplicity, use of metaphor, analogy, and example, multiple forums, repetition, leadership by example, explanation of seeming inconsistencies, and give-and-take. Simplicity serves the dual purposes of ease of dissemination and removal of technical jargon that could confuse and alienate otherwise willing adopters of the change. This is particularly important in the case of AI implementation in radiology, as it requires bringing together people from a variety of backgrounds with differing levels of AI literacy. The use of metaphor, analogy, and example can be an excellent way to avoid jargon while conveying a complex idea in a way that captures attention and persists in memory.

Ensuring that the message is heard, understood, and remembered is also accomplished through two of Kotter's other recommended strategies: the use of multiple forums and repetition. Available forums might include meetings, newsletters, or oppor-

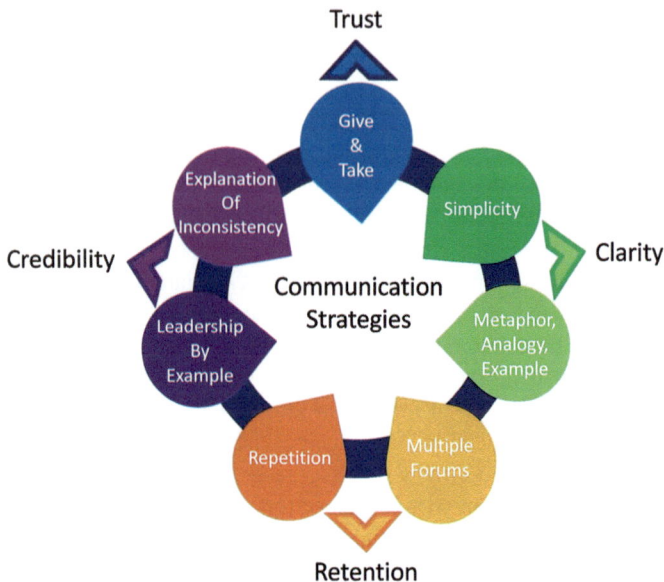

Fig. 4.2 Communication strategies and qualities they foster: trust, clarity, retention, and credibility

tunistic one-to-one conversations. By making a commitment to find opportunities to mention the change vision in routine communication, it becomes easy to communicate repeatedly. Examples include mentioning an article on a new AI solution when a colleague voices a pain point in the reading room or including a brief AI update in a faculty meeting agenda. The many educational opportunities that are available, as discussed in the next section, also serve to demonstrate the vision of the future and establish buy-in.

Establishing and maintaining credibility are essential parts of the communication process, which Kotter argues can be accomplished through leading by example and addressing inconsistencies. When leaders embody the new vision through their actions, it becomes easier for all to trust and follow-suit, particularly skeptics. Addressing seeming inconsistencies with honest explanations that express a desire to improve in the future and reiterating a commitment to the broader goal similarly help to dispense with mistrust.

Last but not least, there is the importance of listening. Offering opportunities for feedback by those being asked to adopt a change makes them feel included while also allowing for the exposure of imperfections in the new system. This not only includes gatekeeping for individual model quality control but also identifying shortcomings in the AI adoption strategy as a whole. Furthermore, in the same way that communication of information by the change leaders should occur in repeated fashion via multiple forums, so should the reception of feedback. The most effective communicators for change will be prepared to receive information any time they are giving it. The credibility and trust that ensues will pay dividends in the long run over the relatively small amount of time and effort that was taken to listen.

4.5 Education Strategies

Among the benefits of an emerging field like AI are the abundance of educational material available and the opportunity for stakeholders across disciplines and career stages to learn together. When seeking out sources of educational content for AI, one need not look far to find a multitude offered by radiology societies including the European Society for Medical Imaging Informatics (EuSoMII), European Society of Radiology (ESR), Society for Imaging Informatics in Medicine (SIIM), Radiological Society of North America (RSNA), and the American College of Radiology (ACR). This content comes in a variety of formats, such as online courses, webinars, AI-focused journals, books, fellowships, online forums, podcasts, and hands-on learning labs at society meetings. Specific examples include the ESR Masterclass in AI, RSNA Radiology: AI Podcasts, EuSoMII webinars, and "EuSoMII on Air" podcasts. A previous booklet in the EuSoMII "Imaging Informatics for Healthcare Professionals" series, entitled, *Introduction to Artificial Intelligence*, offers a concise, entry-level review of foundational AI topics [22]. Individual academic centers and departments may also wish to host their own educational opportunities, which can be beneficial not only to personalize the content to the organization's needs but also to offer a forum for dialogue about the change effort. This could include journal clubs, lecture series, research presentations, focus groups, or panel discussions.

Installing test versions of AI tools and providing demonstrations also afford stakeholders an opportunity to come together to learn about AI and encourage collaboration [5]. By interacting with tools outside of the demands of the clinical environment, learners gain familiarity and trust with the technology at a comfortable pace [5]. This should extend not only to radiologists but also to referring providers, creating another opportunity for cross-disciplinary engagement. The installation of test versions also allows for simulation-based learning, as is recommended by Shafique and colleagues [15]. They propose that this would ideally take the form of simulated "cases" that are integrated into PACS along with the AI model, some in which the AI output is correct and others in which it is incorrect. Through this mechanism, users could not only learn how to use the model within their workflow, but also learn how to identify model failure [15].

Recognizing limitations on the time radiologists can devote to training on AI model use, the above authors propose that simulated cases could appear during the course of a workday on an ongoing basis rather than in bulk. They also suggest that time spent on training modules could be prioritized via tiers based on the clinical impact and time-sensitivity of a model's output. Prioritizing training in this way would require standards governing the amount and type of education required for the use of various models, which the authors suggest should be developed by governing bodies within professional societies. Lastly, they propose that vendors should support the development and distribution of educational content needed for end-user training on their models [15].

4.6 Conclusions

Key aspects of stakeholder engagement with respect to the implementation of AI in radiology include a defined governance structure, cross-disciplinary roles and relationships, open communication, and education. Change leaders should foster an environment that feels welcoming to individuals from diverse educational and career backgrounds, eliminates barriers to involvement, and seeks continuous improvement. This combination of strategy and culture, together with the technological advances afforded by AI, can ensure a brighter future over this next century, in which radiologists are highly visible members of an interconnected health care team.

References

1. Glazer GM, Ruiz-Wibbelsmann JA. The invisible radiologist. Radiology. 2011;258(1):18–22.
2. Kotter J. Leading change. Harvard Business Review Press; 2012.
3. Daye D, Wiggins WF, Lungren MP, Alkasab T, Kottler N, Allen B, Roth CJ, Bizzo BC, Durniak K, Brink JA, Larson DB, Dreyer KJ, Langlotz CP. Implementation of clinical artificial intelligence in radiology: who decides and how? Radiology. 2022;305(1):555–63.
4. Elahi A, Cook TS. Artificial intelligence governance and strategic planning: how we do it. J Am Coll Radiol. 2023;20(9):825–7.
5. Strohm L, Hehakaya C, Ranschaert ER, Boon WP, Moors EH. Implementation of artificial intelligence (AI) applications in radiology: hindering and facilitating factors. Eur Radiol. 2020;30(10):5525–32.
6. Bizzo BC, Dasegowda G, Bridge C, Miller B, Hillis JM, Kalra MK, Durniak K, Stout M, Schultz T, Alkasab T, Dreyer KJ. Addressing the challenges of implementing artificial intelligence tools in clinical practice: principles from experience. J Am Coll Radiol. 2023;20(3):352–60.
7. Kotter E, Ranschaert E. Challenges and solutions for introducing artificial intelligence into daily clinical workflow. Eur Radiol. 2021;31:5–7.
8. Rothenburg S, Gupta S, Bonn W, Kim W. Translation of artificial intelligence into practice: the radiologist as a vendor. J Am Coll Radiol. 2023;20(9):875–6.

9. Haan M, Ongena YP, Hommes S, Kwee TC, Yakar D. A qualitative study to understand patient perspective on the use of artificial intelligence in radiology. J Am Coll Radiol. 2019;16(10):1416–9.

10. Ongena YP, Yakar D, Haan M, Kwee TC. Artificial intelligence in screening mammography: a population survey of women's preferences. J Am Coll Radiol. 2021;18(1):79–86.

11. Kitts AB. Patient perspectives on artificial intelligence in radiology. J Am Coll Radiol. 2023;20(9):863–7.

12. Tyson A, Pasquini G, Spencer A, Funk C. 60% of Americans would be uncomfortable with provider relying on AI in their own healthcare. Pew Research Center; 2023.

13. Hardy M, Harvey H. Artificial intelligence in diagnostic imaging: impact on the radiography profession. Br J Radiol. 2020;93:20190840.

14. HCIAC Corporate Roundtable Subcommittee on Artificial Intelligence. The artificial intelligence era: the role of radiologic technologists and radiation therapists. ASRT Foundation Whitepaper; 2020.

15. Shafique U, Chaudhry US, Towbin AJ. Are the pilots on board? Equipping radiologists for clinical implementation of AI. J Digit Imaging. 2023;36:2329–34.

16. Avanzo M, Trianni A, Botta F, Talamonti C, Stasi M, Iori M. Artificial intelligence and the medical physicist: welcome to the machine. Appl Sci. 2021;11:1–17.

17. Zanca F, Hernandez-Giron I, Avanzo M, Guidi G, Crijns W, Diaz O, Kagadis GC, Rampado O, Lønne PI, Ken S, Colgan N, Zaidi H, Zakaria GA, Kortesniemi M. Expanding the medical physicist curricular and professional programme to include artificial intelligence. Eur J Med Phys. 2021;83:174–83.

18. Andersson J, Nyholm T, Ceberg C, Almen A, Bernhardt P, Fransson A, Olsson LE. Artificial intelligence and the medical physics profession—a Swedish perspective. Eur J Med Phys. 2021;88:218–25.

19. Shrestha RB. Roles and relationships in healthcare. In: Branstetter B, editor. Practical imaging informatics: foundations and applications for medical imaging. 2nd ed. Springer; 2021. p. 229–48.

20. Ranschaert E, Topff L, Pianykh O. Optimization of radiology workflow with artificial intelligence. Radiol Clin North Am. 2021;59:955–66.

21. AI for imaging—Feasibility project in practice of a national infrastructure for the application of artificial intelligence (AI) products for radiology. 2023. https://radiologen.nl/secties/techniek/aifi

22. Klontzas ME, Fanni SC, Neri E. Introduction to artificial intelligence. Springer International Publishing AG; 2023.

Exploring and Assessing AI Models

5

Peter M. A. van Ooijen and Sergey Morozov

Key Points
- The assessment of AI models in healthcare is a critical process that demands meticulous attention to ensure efficacy, safety, and regulatory compliance.
- Stakeholders from academia, professional societies, industry, and government play a vital role in developing and implementing frameworks and models for the validation of AI solutions in healthcare settings.
- Transparency, accountability, and continuous quality assurance are essential pillars for the successful integration and utilization of AI-driven initiatives in the complex healthcare landscape.

P. M. A. van Ooijen (✉)
Department of Radiotherapy, University Medical Center Groningen, Groningen, The Netherlands
e-mail: p.m.a.van.ooijen@umcg.nl

S. Morozov
European Society of Medical Imaging Informatics, Liege, Belgium
e-mail: smorozov@post.harvard.edu

© The Author(s), under exclusive license to Springer Nature Switzerland AG 2024
E. Ranschaert et al. (eds.), *AI Implementation in Radiology*, Imaging Informatics for Healthcare Professionals,
https://doi.org/10.1007/978-3-031-68942-0_5

5.1   Introduction

The selection and evaluation of AI solutions play a crucial role in change management. This involves assessing different AI models, products, software platforms, or commercial solutions available in the market. Key considerations include accuracy, reliability, scalability, regulatory compliance, integration capabilities, and the potential impact on workflow and patient care. To enable such selection, evaluation, monitoring, and quality assurance (QA), new systems will have to be developed and deployed and new positions for people with special skills will have to be created to manage AI solutions. Furthermore, tools such as the Integration the Healthcare Enterprise (IHE) integration profiles are needed for the integration of all functional systems and to orchestrate the functions of several AI models.

When exploring and assessing AI models for their merit to healthcare, we must focus on different types of validation [1]. First, **methodological validation** of a developed model needs to be performed to establish the performance of the model in terms of accuracy, robustness, reproducibility, and generalizability. This performance must be assessed using carefully collected and curated retrospective datasets that closely resemble the data as it will be used in the clinical deployment of the model. Second, **clinical validation** of the tool is needed, which not only includes prospective analysis of the model's performance, but also determination of the clinical value of the model within the workflow in which it will be used. This clinical value can include value to the patient, to the radiologist using the AI and also other physicians.

When moving to actual implementation of the AI solutions in clinical practice, we should also have an extensive analysis of the solution including information about published results of clinical trials, Medical Device Regulation (MDR) related materials, information about security and General Data Protection Regulation (GDPR) compliance (Data Privacy Impact Analysis—DPIA, for more information, see Chap. 6 on legal and ethical aspects of AI in radiology), and interoperability information. Additionally teaching and training materials for the users should be available to allow them to properly use the provided AI solutions.

In this chapter, we first look into the assessment of pre-deployment performance. These are things to consider during the development and testing of a new AI model in order to ensure sufficient performance. The main responsibility for this part lies with the developer of the model. Next, we look at post-deployment performance. This concerns the selection and acceptance of AI models in clinical settings as well as user-satisfaction and long-term quality assurance. Here the responsibility is extended to the organization implementing and using the AI model. Finally, various rules and regulations, integration profiles, and assessment frameworks are discussed. These are important guides and tools for the assessment of both pre- and post-deployment performance.

5.2   Assessment of Pre-deployment Performance

When building an AI tool, its pre-deployment performance is tested during the development cycle. This involves the training and test (or validation) phase. For this purpose, the dataset is split into a training and validation set, for use in the training phase and the testing phase, respectively. The training set is used to train the AI model, while the testing set is used to evaluate its pre-deployment performance on previously unseen data. This determines if the model is accurate and reliable. Model scalability can contain several aspects. For example, a scalable model should be able to handle increasing amounts of data without a significant decrease in performance, it should show improved performance with more computational resources, and it should have low latency and high-throughput during inference. If possible, it is recommended to use a dataset for the test phase from another source as the training phase to enable the assessment of the generalizability of a model, and to avoid the presence of any bias from the training data in performing those validation measurements.

5.2.1   Model Performance

One of the primary factors to evaluate in AI solutions is accuracy. Accuracy refers to how well an AI model performs in delivering the desired outcomes. The ability of an AI solution to make correct predictions or classifications is crucial for its reliability and effectiveness.

Besides sensitivity and specificity, which are commonly used in healthcare, various other statistical metrics are used to assess the performance of AI models, such as precision, recall, and F1 score. Precision measures the ratio of correctly predicted positive instances to the total predicted positive instances. Recall, which is the same as sensitivity, measures the ratio of correctly predicted positive instances to the total actual positive instances. The F1 score combines precision and recall providing a balanced measure of accuracy. These metrics help measure the model's ability to correctly classify or predict data.

By evaluating performance, we can determine the reliability of an AI solution and its suitability for specific tasks. However, it is important to note that achieving 100% accuracy in real-world scenarios is often not feasible. Therefore, AI solutions should be evaluated based on domain-specific requirements and benchmarks rather than aiming for perfect accuracy.

5.2.2   Reliability

Reliability is another crucial aspect to consider when evaluating AI solutions. It refers to the consistency and dependability of a model's performance. An AI solution must not only be accurate, but also remain reliable in different situations and scenarios, such as incomplete data and data noise. With respect to reliability, the term generalizability is also often used, referring to the ability of a model trained in a local dataset to be also effectively used in datasets obtained from other sources (e.g., data obtained from different geographical locations).

To assess reliability (or robustness), rigorous testing and validation procedures are necessary. This involves subjecting the AI solution to various challenging scenarios to evaluate its performance under adverse conditions. It helps identify potential weaknesses, vulnerabilities, or biases that may affect the reliability of the AI solution. This testing can involve selection of a dataset from another source, introducing perturbations in the input data, simulating data from different distributions, or evaluating the AI solution's performance on edge cases.

Furthermore, monitoring the performance of AI solutions over time in a real-world environment is essential to ensure their continued reliability. AI models can degrade or become less accurate over time due to data drift (where the input to the models changes) or concept drift (where the underlying data distribution changes). Monitoring of the input data to the AI model and regular retraining and monitoring of the AI solution itself can help detect and address these changes, ensuring the AI model reliability and effectiveness in the long run.

5.2.3 Scalability

Scalability refers to an AI solution's ability to handle increasing data volume and workload without sacrificing its performance. As organizations generate and accumulate large amounts of data, it is crucial to assess the scalability of AI solutions to ensure their viability in real-world scenarios especially in those settings in the clinical field where time is a crucial component.

Evaluating scalability involves considering factors such as the model's efficiency in processing large amounts of data, the availability of computational resources, and the system's ability to scale horizontally or vertically. Horizontal scalability refers to the capability of distributing the workload across multiple machines or nodes, while vertical scalability refers to increasing the computational power or resources of a single machine.

AI solutions can be evaluated based on their scalability by analyzing their performance under different workload sizes and data volumes. Stress testing, which involves pushing the AI solution to its limits by increasing the workload or data volume, can provide insights into its scalability capabilities. Evaluating resource utilization and the ability to handle concurrent requests is also important in assessing scalability.

Scalability assessment ensures that the AI solution can handle future growth and accommodate the expanding needs of the organization. It allows organizations to make informed decisions about scaling their AI infrastructure and avoiding performance bottlenecks.

5.3   Assessment of Post-deployment Performance

Although the pre-deployment performance measures will give insight into the usability of the model, it does not always map directly to the post-deployment performance of the same model. Often the post-deployment performance is not only dependent on the pre-deployment performance of the model but also on, for example, the role and position of the model in the clinical workflow. Assessing the impact of AI solutions on workflow and patient care is therefore essential. It involves evaluating how well the AI solution optimizes workflows, enhances efficiency, and improves patient care outcomes. The successful integration of AI solutions into the clinical process (interoperability) can lead to significant improvements in productivity, accuracy, and decision-making processes.

5.4   Impact on Workflow and Patient Care

To assess the impact on workflow, organizations should evaluate the AI solution's compatibility with existing processes and systems. It involves understanding the current workflow, identifying potential bottlenecks or inefficiencies, and assessing how the AI solution can streamline or automate certain tasks. User feedback, workflow analysis, and process mapping can provide valuable insights into the impact of AI solutions on workflow optimization.

Patient care assessment focuses on evaluating the AI solution's ability to improve clinical outcomes and enhance patient experiences. This assessment involves examining the accuracy and reliability of AI predictions or diagnoses and their impact on treatment decisions. It is essential to consider the AI solution's impact on patient safety, care coordination, and overall healthcare delivery. It is also important to evaluate here the impact on the users themselves. How do they value and use the AI models' outcome? Related risks are, for example, automation bias, overreliance, and deskilling.

Automation bias refers to the tendency of humans to favor decisions made by automated systems because of this users might overtrust the AI model's predictions and ignore other information, leading to potential errors.

Overreliance is when users depend too heavily on the AI model, to the point where they stop using their own judgment or skills.

Deskilling refers to the loss or degradation of human skills. If users rely on AI models too much and do not practice their own skills, they may find those skills deteriorating over time.

These risks could lead to a decrease in diagnostic accuracy or even loss of skills which renders the user unable to still assess the validity of an AI model outcome. Therefore, it is important to design AI systems that support human decision-making without encouraging overdependence maintaining the balance where the AI model serves as a tool to augment human skills, rather than to replace them.

Evaluating the impact on workflow and patient care should involve stakeholders from different domains, including clinicians, administrators, and end users. Their perspectives and feedback can help assess the practical implications and potential benefits of implementing AI solutions in healthcare settings or other relevant industries. Important to consider here is that the actual clinical impact might be difficult to measure and could require the integration of data from different domains. For example, the radiological report might be considered the gold standard to evaluate the clinical performance of an AI model. However, the validity of this gold standard could be doubted since information about the clinical outcome might be obtained later, for example, through histology or surgery.

5.5 Regulatory Compliance

AI solutions used in a healthcare setting often deal with sensitive data and have ethical and legal implications. Regulatory compliance is crucial to ensure that AI solutions adhere to relevant laws, regulations, and ethical standards. Organizations must assess the compliance of AI solutions to mitigate risks and maintain trust among stakeholders.

When assessing regulatory compliance, several aspects need to be considered. Data privacy and security measures are of utmost importance to protect personal information and ensure confidentiality. For this, compliance with regulations such as the General Data Protection Regulation (GDPR) in the European Union, or the Health Insurance Portability and Accountability Act (HIPAA) in the United States, is essential. It is also important to ensure that AI solutions handle and store data securely, with appropriate access controls and encryption techniques.

Transparency in decision-making processes is another aspect of regulatory compliance. Understanding how AI solutions make predictions or decisions is crucial for accountability and fairness. Explainable AI methods, such as rule-based systems or transparent machine learning models, can help provide insights into the reasoning behind AI decisions. Assessing the transparency and interpretability of AI solutions is necessary to comply with regulatory requirements and build trust with end users and stakeholders. However, although mechanisms exist to provide some insight in their decision process, the explainability of more complex AI solutions such as those using deep learning or generative models is still a major challenge.

Organizations should also consider ethical implications when assessing AI solutions. Bias assessment and mitigation are critical to ensure fair treatment and prevent discrimination. Evaluating whether AI solutions perpetuate or amplify biases in the data or decision-making process is essential. AI solutions should be designed and assessed with fairness and equity in mind. In their final recommendations for integration of AI into radiological practice, Recht et al. state that "Guidelines for the ethical use of imaging AI need to be developed and radiologists in combination with ethicists should lead this effort" [1]. More information about the legal and ethical aspects of AI in radiology can be found in Chap. 6.

5.6 Integration Capabilities

AI solutions need to seamlessly integrate with existing systems and workflows within an organization. Evaluating integration capabilities involves assessing whether the AI solution is compatible with the organization's infrastructure. Interoperability, the ability of different systems to exchange and interpret data seamlessly is also a significant consideration. Healthcare data standards, such as DICOM (Digital Imaging and Communication in Medicine) and HL7 (Health Level Seven), ensure interoperability by defining how data should be structured and exchanged. Furthermore, Integrating the Healthcare Enterprise (IHE) is developing integration profiles to help developers and customers to ensure optimal interoperability of AI with other systems already in the clinical workflow. These are described in the IHE Radiology white paper on AI interoperability that was published in 2021 [18]. Assessing the AI solution's compliance with those relevant data standards and its ability to integrate with other systems based on these standards is essential for successful integration.

Integration assessment begins with understanding the organization's existing systems, databases, and data formats. It involves evaluating how well the AI solution can interact with these systems and whether it requires any modifications or additional software components for integration. Compatibility with programming languages, databases, and data exchange protocols should be considered.

The availability and effectiveness of APIs (application programming interfaces) are crucial in assessing integration capabilities. An API is a set of rules and protocols that allows one software application to interact with another. It defines the methods and data formats that applications can use to request and exchange information. APIs allow different software systems to communicate and share data effectively. Evaluating the quality, flexibility, and functionality of APIs provided by the AI solution or the platform it is built upon can help determine its integration capabilities.

5.7   Assessment Frameworks and Models

Assessment frameworks and models for AI play a crucial role in ensuring the responsible and ethical development, deployment, and use of artificial intelligence systems. They provide a structured approach to evaluate various aspects of AI applications, fostering transparency, accountability, and trust in the technology.

The FDA has issued guidelines for Good Machine Learning Practice [2]. They looked at the entire process from development to roll-out and live monitoring. Emphasis is placed on a culture of quality and organizational excellence in the development of AI applications. As soon as the system is ready to be used in practice, a pre-market proof of the safety and effectiveness of the system is requested. A review of the Software as a Medical Device specifications and an adjustment protocol for the model is also required. After this, continuous monitoring is required when using an artificial intelligence system. This monitoring can also be used to collect data to improve the system. Although all these steps seem logical, their practical implementation is complicated, and it is not yet completely clear how specific steps should be implemented.

To put these kinds of principles into practice to perform assessment of AI solutions, various frameworks and models have been developed by academia, professional societies, industry, and government [3]. In the following sections, we will show some examples of those frameworks and models without the illusion of being complete.

5.7.1 Academia/Professional Societies

Academia and professional societies are often in the forefront of new technological development and therefore the call for frameworks and models often starts there.

This need for proper assessment of AI in academia starts with standardized reporting on the development of AI. Guidelines for manuscripts dealing with AI implementation and validation such as the Checklist for Artificial Intelligence in Medical Imaging (CLAIM) help to standardize reporting [4]. Recht et al. state in their recommendations that "For the responsible introduction of AI in clinical practice, proper validation strategies are essential. A way forward is to link AI use cases as defined by the clinical end users (including labeled data) to challenges designed to objectively assess and compare model performance" [1].

Frameworks have also been developed to evaluate commercial AI solutions for their responsible use and value in clinical practice. For example, the Canadian Association of Radiologists published their AI validation and evaluation framework [5]. It facilitates dialogue with the AI software industry and equips healthcare leaders and radiologists with tools to evaluate the suitability of AI software. The suggested software assessment framework establishes the basis for a radiologist-driven prospective validation network of radiology AI software. Morozov et al. [6] published a comprehensive evaluation methodology for AI services. They propose to assess user experience, accessibility, safety, and diagnostic accuracy of such AI services using an independent reference dataset. Furthermore, Omoumi et al. have developed a checklist for radiology AI models and have developed the "ECLAIR" guidelines for evaluation AI models in radiology before purchase [7].

Dedicated reporting cards are also developed to provide insight into the possible use of an AI model in clinical practice. Sendak et al. [8] prove the Model Facts labels that are advocated to present machine learning model information to clinical end users. Similarly, Richards et al. [9] propose AI FactSheets to achieve higher quality and more consistent AI documentation to address ethical and legal concerns and general social impacts of AI systems.

5.7.2   Industry

Companies active in the field of artificial intelligence also need standardized frameworks and models to help assess their applications [3]. Similar to the examples from Sendak and Richards, they also develop standard reporting tools for both datasets used for training and testing AI, and for the AI models themselves. Examples of this are the Datasheets for Datasets as developed by Microsoft [10, 11]. To describe AI models, Google has developed Model Cards [12], and IBM has developed Factsheets [13].

These frameworks and models provide very practical tools to give in-depth information about a dataset used to train and test an AI model and about the model itself. To this end, a datasheet typically provides information about motivation for data collection, composition of the dataset, collection process, performed cleaning and preprocessing steps, labeling, use, and distribution and maintenance of the data collection. A model card will provide information about the developer of the model, the intended use, the validation and performance metrics, the training and test data used, and the use recommendations and warnings. In most cases, these models are published as open science contributions, and thus can be used freely. Despite that, unfortunately, there is not yet a widespread adoption of those approaches in healthcare AI.

5.7.3   Government

More practical tools have also been developed by governmental organizations, sometimes in co-creation with academia.

To develop guidelines based on the concerns and specific ethical issues with AI, the European Commission decided to form an independent high-level experts' group on AI in 2018 to work on Ethical Guidelines for trustworthy AI. This resulted in a report and an assessment list for trustworthy artificial intelligence, ALTAI.

The report defines a framework for trustworthy AI which they subdivide into lawful AI, ethical AI, and robust AI. The foundations of trustworthy AI are to adhere to ethical principles based on fundamental rights. To achieve this, four ethical principles are defined: respect for human autonomy, prevention of harm, fairness, and explicability. To realize trustworthy AI based on those foundations, seven key requirements are introduced:

1. Human agency and oversight.
2. Technical robustness and safety.
3. Privacy and data governance.
4. Transparency.
5. Diversity, non-discrimination, and fairness.
6. Societal and environmental well-being.
7. Accountability.

The aim is to evaluate and address these 7 key requirements continuously through an AI system's life cycle via both technical and non-technical methods. It is important to state here that all seven requirements defined are of equal importance, support each other, and should be implemented and evaluated throughout the AI system's life cycle.

To support the actual implementation of the ethical guidelines for trustworthy AI, the European Committee provides the ALTAI assessment list that can be used for self-assessment of a specific AI tool against the seven ethics guidelines for trustworthy AI [17]. After free registration to the site, you can define an AI tool to evaluate and during the ALTAI process you will be guided through the seven requirements and must provide answers to several questions per requirement. Based on the answers, an analysis of your AI tool is performed that results in a plot that shows how well the tool adheres to the seven requirements allowing to evaluate which items require more attention to obtain a trustworthy AI solution. Besides this analysis, the tool will also provide concrete recommendations for improvement.

Another example of such a practical tool is the Innovation Funnel for Valuable AI in Healthcare developed by the University Medical Center in Utrecht in the Netherlands and adopted by the Ministry of Health, Welfare, and Sport [14]. This Innovation

Funnel helps researchers and developers in the process from development to scaling up valuable artificial intelligence (AI). It offers clues in the scope for action within the laws and regulations by supporting the innovation process in five domains: value, application, ethics, technology, and responsibility. The Innovation Funnel can be downloaded from the ministry website.

Finally, in the European AI Act will also have a major effect on the way we develop, implement, and validate AI tools in the clinical domain. While the actual effect of the AI Act on the implementation of AI in clinical practice is still somewhat unclear, there is one element that will definitely have an impact in the healthcare sector, namely that suppliers/industry will also face liability with regard to AI tools, not just the radiologist as has been the case to date.

5.8 Discussion

At this moment, we unfortunately still see limited scientific evidence of clinical impact and performance of AI. This kind of evidence should come from large prospective multicenter trials, but they prove to be difficult to set up and fund. One reason for this is the large number of different tools that are available on the market and that should individually be tested. Furthermore, developments are fast and models are retrained and updated frequently. Therefore, more centralized controlled trials that allow parallel assessment of multiple tools would need to be implemented. Although this will be difficult, obtaining proof of clinical impact and performance of AI is crucial for increasing the acceptance rate of AI tools for clinical practice.

We must be aware that the assessment of AI tools does not stop at the acquisition or commissioning of a new tool in clinical practice. After successful implementation and integration of AI into clinical practice, there is a need for continuous evaluation and real-world performance monitoring [15]. This also involves extending the methodologies described in this chapter to also come to the implementation of quality assurance (QA) approaches for AI solutions since regulatory approval is not sufficient for the safe and effective use of AI in the local setting [16].

Because of the novelty of AI solutions in clinical practice, effective training of staff involved in installation and deployment and of the end-user is crucial for successful adoption. Although not covered in detail in this chapter, it would be a point of concern when assessing a solution for use in clinical practice to make sure that proper training materials are provided by the vendor of the system. To assess this, the level of support provided by a vendor during implementation, deployment, and maintenance should be assessed as well as the availability of training resources and ongoing assistance. Besides this another aspect to consider is the reliability of the software provider in the immature AI market of the current day. This involves the vendor reputation and stability. Relevant aspects to investigate are the vendor's track record, financial stability, customer satisfaction, and their commitment to long-term support and updates.

5.9   Conclusions

The assessment of AI solutions plays a vital role in change management. By considering accuracy, reliability, scalability, regulatory compliance, integration capabilities, impact on workflow and patient care, as well as the need for management functions and integration tools, organizations can make informed decisions about adopting and implementing AI solutions. Continuous assessment and improvement are essential to ensure the effectiveness and long-term success of AI-driven initiatives. For this, solid infrastructure and adapted policy are necessary, so that feedback can be provided and evaluated, not only from the group of users (radiologists and others) but also from the referring clinicians and other recipients of the results. Acknowledging that the ground truth for patient outcomes may not come from the radiologist but rather from a surgical pathology result or clinical/biochemical information obtained after treatment is also important. This will require integration of multiple other data in the feedback loop, which is still a challenge. As technology continues to evolve, organizations must remain vigilant in assessing and adapting their AI solutions to meet emerging challenges and opportunities.

References

1. Recht MP, Dewey M, Dreyer K, Langlotz C, Niessen W, Prainsack B, Smith JJ. Integrating artificial intelligence into the clinical practice of radiology: challenges and recommendations. Eur Radiol. 2020;30:3576–84.
2. https://www.fda.gov/medical-devices/software-medical-device-samd/good-machine-learning-practice-medical-device-development-guiding-principles. Accessed 5 Feb 2024.
3. De Biase A, Sourlos N, van Ooijen PMA. Standardization of artificial intelligence development in radiotherapy. Semin Radiat Oncol. 2022;32:415–20.
4. Mongan J, Moy L, Kahn CE. Checklist for artificial intelligence in medical imaging (CLAIM): a guide for authors and reviewers. Radiology. 2020;2:e200029.
5. Tanguay W, Acar P, Fine B, Abdollel M, Gong B, Cadrin-Chenevert A, Chartrand-Lefebvre C, Chalaoui J, Gorgos A, Shu-Lei Chin A, Prenovault J, Guilbert F, Letourneau-Guillon L, Chong J, Tang A. Assessment of radiology artificial intelligence software: a validation and evaluation framework. Can Assoc Radiol J. 2023;74(2):326–33.
6. Morozov SP, Gombolevskiy VA, Blokhin IA, Semenov SS, Logunova TA, Andreychenko AE. A comprehensive evaluation methodology for the publicly accessible AI services for medical diagnostics. medRxiv. 2021.
7. Omoumi P, Ducarouge A, Tournier A, Hm H, Kahn CE Jr, Louvet-de Verchere F, Pinto dos Santos D, Kober T, Richiardi J. To buy or not to buy—evaluating commercial AI solutions in radiology (the ÉCLAIR guidelines). Eur Radiol. 2021;31:37863796.
8. Sendak MP, Gao M, Brajer N, et al. Presenting machine learning model information to clinical end users with model fact labels. NPJ Digit Med. 2020;3:41. https://doi.org/10.1038/s41746-020-0253-3.
9. Richards J, Piorkowski D, Hind M, et al. A methodology for creating AI FactSheets. arXiv. https://arxiv.org/abs/2006.13796. Accessed 5 Feb 2024.
10. Gebru T, Morgenstern J, Vecchione B, Wortman Vaughan J, Wallach H, Daume H III, Crawford K. Datasheets for datasets. Arxiv:1803.09010. Last revised 1 Dec 2021.
11. Crawford K, Daume H III, Vorvoreanu M, et al. Datasheets for datasets. Microsoft. https://www.microsoft.com/enus/research/project/datasheets-for-datasets/. Accessed 10 Nov 2021.

12. Mitchell M, Wu S, Zeldivar A, et al. Model cards for model reporting. 2019. https://arxiv.org/abs/1810.03993. Accessed 10 Nov 2021.
13. Arnold M, Bellamy R, Hind M, et al. FactSheets: increasing trust in AI services through supplier's declarations of conformity. IBM J Res & Dev. 2019;63:6–1. https://doi.org/10.1147/JRD.2019.2942288.
14. https://www.datavoorgezondheid.nl/documenten/publicaties/2021/07/15/innovation-funnel-for-valuable-ai-in-healthcare. Accessed 5 Feb 2024.
15. Allen B, Dreyer K, Stibolt R, Agarwal S, Coombs L, Treml C, Elkholy M, Brink L, Wald C. Evaluation and real-world performance monitoring of artificial intelligence models in clinical practice: try it, buy it, check it. J Am Coll Radiol. 2021;18:1489–96.
16. Lundstrom C, Lindvall M. Mapping the landscape of care providers' quality assurance approaches for AI in diagnostic imaging. J Digit Imaging. 2023;36:379–87.
17. https://altai.insight-centre.org/. Accessed 5 Feb 2024.
18. Genereaux B, O'Donnell K, Bialecki B, Diedrich K, Roth CJ, Schroeder A, Tenenholtz N, Younis K, Zachmann H, the IHE Radiology Community. IHE Radiology White Paper AI Interoperability in Imaging. IHE_RAD_White_Paper_AI_Interoperability_in_Imaging_Rev1-1_Pub_2021-10-12. Accessed 12 Apr 2024.

Legal and Ethical Aspects of AI in Radiology

6

Bart Custers and Eduard Fosch-Villaronga

Key Points
- Legal and ethical considerations are essential for the successful deployment of AI in radiology beyond mere technological and medical concerns.
- Compliance with legal norms is mandatory to avoid illegal practices, covering safety, privacy, security, and non-discrimination in AI applications.
- Ethical aspects like human dignity, autonomy, and accountability are crucial, especially where legal guidelines are absent or ambiguous.
- The relevance of legal and ethical aspects can vary by context, requiring different sets of considerations for each AI application.
- Impact assessments and value-sensitive design are effective methods for identifying and integrating legal and ethical considerations into AI development.

B. Custers (✉) · E. Fosch-Villaronga
eLaw Center for Law and Digital Technologies, Leiden University,
Leiden, Zuid-Holland, The Netherlands
e-mail: b.h.m.custers@law.leidenuniv.nl;
e.fosch.villaronga@law.leidenuniv.nl

© The Author(s), under exclusive license to Springer Nature
Switzerland AG 2024
E. Ranschaert et al. (eds.), *AI Implementation in Radiology*, Imaging
Informatics for Healthcare Professionals,
https://doi.org/10.1007/978-3-031-68942-0_6

6.1   Introduction

The use of AI in radiology offers many opportunities, mainly because AI tools are very good at dealing with large amounts of data and recognizing patterns and singularities, i.e., unique or unusual patterns in the data that might not be immediately apparent or easily recognizable by human observers [1]. Since radiology deals with large amounts of data, such as medical images, clinical data, and radiopharmaceutical data, AI tools can help with fast and efficient processing and analysis of such data and assist radiologists and other medical experts in determining diagnoses and potential treatments. AI can also discover new patterns that are previously unknown or detect singularities that human observers may easily overlook [2]. Obviously, and rightfully so, the focus on the successful use of AI in radiology is on both technological aspects (ensuring the technology works and offers added value) and medical aspects (making sure patients benefit from this).

However, developing, implementing, and deploying AI in radiology require more than focusing only on these technological and medical aspects. To ensure basic levels of user-friendliness, user acceptance, and support from both patients and the public, it is essential also to consider legal and ethical aspects [3]. Legal requirements are a conditio sine qua non: non-compliance with legal norms would constitute an illegal practice. Laws and regulations are sometimes considered barriers to innovation, as they constitute complicating factors hindering the liberty of developers in realizing their visions. Sometimes laws and regulations are not considered at all, simply because people developing new technologies have different, non-legal backgrounds and are unaware of legal obligations, let alone how to implement them [4]. Nevertheless, legal rules are rules of the game that need to be considered by any party, as these rules are set to protect people, most notably patients, from practices and technologies that could be potentially harmful to them. As such, these rules should not be seen as barriers to innovation but as incentives to realize better innovation. Considering legal aspects is not only mandatory, but it can also yield technology with higher levels of safety, user-friendliness, user acceptance, and public support [5].

The same applies to ethical norms. These rules may be softer, as there is no legal obligation (and no sanction) to observe ethical norms. Contrary to legal norms, ethical norms cannot be enforced in courts. Nevertheless, ethical norms may need to be considered in cases with no legal requirements, which is often the case when dealing with new technologies. For instance, when dealing with AI, the EU has enacted the AI Act[1] [6], but this legislation is not yet immediately fully effective. Until then, it depends on ethical norms whether actors already take the future legal norms into account. Even when legislation is in place, such legislation often offers ambiguous or insufficient guidance. When legal norms are absent or unclear, examining the underlying ethical norms is necessary for further guidance.

This chapter examines the most relevant legal and ethical aspects of AI in radiology. This overview is not exhaustive; other legal and ethical aspects may also be relevant depending on the context. Therefore, this chapter also offers approaches that can be used to identify and qualify legal and ethical aspects further. Early identification of legal and ethical issues will help avoid or mitigate the risks they pose [7]. Legal and ethical aspects can be transformed into legal and ethical design requirements, allowing to consider these aspects in the design of new technologies, making them inherently compliant and safe [8].

This chapter is structured as follows. Section 6.2 examines the most relevant legal aspects in the context of AI in radiology: safety, privacy and data protection, security, and bias and non-discrimination. Section 6.3 examines the most pertinent ethical aspects linked to these developments: human dignity, autonomy, and accountability. Section 6.4 discusses approaches, most notably, impact assessments and value-sensitive design, that can be used to more comprehensively identify legal and ethical aspects more comprehensively and subsequently take them into account for AI in radiology. Section 6.5 offers conclusions.

---

[1]The AI Act entered into force on August 1, 2024. However, it will take effect in stages, with some provisions coming into effect sooner than others. For example, prohibitions on certain AI systems and requirements for AI literacy will apply from February 2025, while the requirements for general-purpose AI models will apply from August 2025. Most provisions in the AI Act will apply after a two-year implementation period (i.e. from 1 August 2026).

6.2   Legal Aspects

This section examines the most relevant legal aspects for AI in radiology. These are safety, privacy and data protection, security, and bias and non-discrimination respectively.

6.2.1   Safety

AI systems have occasionally made sensational headlines for self-driving cars misclassifying snowmen as pedestrians or algorithms in social media misclassifying men for women [9, 10]. However, misclassification in safety-critical domains like healthcare can lead to significant harm [11–13]. Think, for instance, about spurious correlations, which refer to statistical associations between features and labels that exhibit predictive efficacy within the training distribution but do not maintain this predictive power in the test distribution. Using background color for object recognition, which led to confusing huskies with wolves [14] in the past or the reliance on surgical markers for medical diagnostics are examples that could lead to fatal outcomes [15].

From the perspective of ensuring AI safety, the optimal scenario involves developing a sophisticated AI system that allows us to harness its computational advantages while maintaining adequate and meaningful control [16]. Still, continuous budgetary pressures push for removing the human out of the equation in AI-driven healthcare, which is problematic [17, 18]. Indeed, while recent advances in deep learning, particularly in radiology, offer potential benefits such as cost reduction and increased efficiency, automating human cognitive processes through AI introduces new risks for safety [19]. An FDA-approved system developed by IDx is an automated diagnostic system that can independently assess images of the back of the eye for signs of diabetic eye disease [20]. It operates at or above the level of a human expert, potentially eliminating the need for human intervention in diagnosis and treatment decisions. This advancement enables non-eye care healthcare providers to utilize the system for screening decisions and basic treatment plans, bypassing the involvement of clinicians. Such automation introduces risks, such as overdiagnosing eye disease, leading to unnecessary referrals and increased healthcare costs, or underdiagnosing, resulting in undertreatment and preventable blindness [21].

In this respect, the AI High-Level Expert Group on AI in 2019 recognized the critical role of technical robustness in achieving trustworthy AI [22] and preventing harm [23, 24]. While these recommendations struggle with practical implementation, lessons could be drawn from industries that have successfully enhanced safety but also faced failures, such as the aviation industry [25]. The first lesson emphasizes the need to consider AI system failures independently of their intended purpose, demanding proactive identification and mitigation of potential risks [26]. The second lesson underscores meticulous implementation and testing, treating AI algorithms, input, and output with equal care. Ensuring AI systems detect and communicate inconsistencies or errors in inputs is crucial [27]. The third lesson highlights the necessity of notifying and training individuals involved in workflows incorporating AI systems, even for those expected to be transparent.

These lessons learned highlight that, while technical solutions are essential, they alone may not be enough to guarantee safety. Ensuring that secure algorithms are effectively implemented in real-world systems and preventing the deployment of unsafe systems may necessitate additional socio technical measures and institutions [28].

6.2.2 Privacy and Data Protection

Privacy is a human right enshrined in legal instruments, intended to allow people to shield themselves or their information from others. Traditionally, privacy was focused on the home and family life, such as Article 8 of the European Convention on Human Rights (ECHR) and Article 7 of the EU Charter on fundamental rights (CFR). Privacy also includes protection of personal communication, such as letters and phone calls. Bodily privacy refers to bodily integrity, which can also be relevant in the context of radiology, as tools and instruments in radiology can be invasive to the human body. With the rise of information technology, informational privacy, also referred to as data privacy, is gaining importance. Informational privacy focuses on personal data intrusions, including unauthorized access to personal data or unlawful processing of personal data.

The CFR contains a fundamental right to data protection, unique in the world, that focuses on the protection of personal data. The EU General Data Protection Regulation (GDPR) elaborates on this fundamental right by setting rules for the collection and processing of personal data. Typically, the GDPR prescribes that the processing has to be lawful, fair, and transparent (Article 5.1 GDPR). The purposes for which the data are collected and processed have to be stated in advance (purpose specification) and the data may not be used for other purposes (purpose or use limitation) and data may only be collected and processed when necessary for these purposes (collection limitation or data minimization). Data has to be accurate and up to date (data quality). When data is no longer necessary, it has to be removed (storage limitation). The data needs to be processed in a way that ensures appropriate security and has to be protected against unlawful processing, accidental loss, destruction, and damage (data integrity, confidentiality). Furthermore, the data controller is responsible for compliance (accountability, Article 5.2 GDPR).

Processing is only lawful when the data subject has given consent, when the processing of the data is necessary for the performance of a contract (e.g., an agreement between doctor and patient), when the processing is necessary for compliance with a legal obligation (usually for law enforcement purposes) or any of the other legal bases in Article 6 GDPR. The processing of sensitive data such as personal data revealing ethnicity, political or religious beliefs, genetic data, or data concerning sexual orientation is not allowed, unless exceptions apply (Article 9 GDPR).

According to the GDPR, data subjects have several rights regarding their personal data, including a right to transparent information on the data collected and the purposes for which it is processed (Article 12–14 GDPR), a right to access their data (Article 15 GDPR), a right to rectification (Article 16 GDPR), a right to erasure (Article 17 GDPR), and a right not to be subject to automated decision-making (Article 22 GDPR).

When using any AI tools in radiology, it is therefore important to be transparent toward patients and others whose data are being processed. Data subjects should always be informed about which data on them is collected and processed, for which purposes, and how this may affect them. In most cases, the most suitable legal basis for processing the data is consent, which should be informed consent [29]. If the use of AI tools results in automated decisions on patients, patients should be informed about their right not to be subject to this. If people invoke this right under Article 22 GDPR, their data should be excluded from datasets processed by the AI tools. Although this right is rarely invoked, it should be noted that if many people would invoke this right, it could significantly bias the results that AI tools yield if data is used for training purposes. For processing data as part of clinical practice, patients should be informed if results are obtained by means of AI analysis. This transparency obligation can be realized, for example, by using disclaimers in the provided report stating that results (e.g., measurements) are provided by AI [30]. Such a disclaimer could also regulate any ambiguity that might arise when radiologists provide other suggestions that differ from that of the AI, whereas such a disclaimer can state that the result of the radiologist is considered to be the leading result of the report and overrides the AI result [31].

6.2.3   Security

Integrating deep learning algorithms into clinical systems for tasks like diagnosis introduces susceptibility to manipulation or hacking through adversarial attacks, even when there is human supervision. Although researchers claim that there has been no well-known attack [32], hacking AI in radiology could pose a risk to patient safety and the accuracy of medical decisions, impacting the overall quality of healthcare [33]. If AI systems used in radiology get hacked, it could lead to severe problems. Imagine a situation where AI helps doctors make important decisions about their health based on medical images, like X-rays or MRIs [34]. Hackers who interfere with this system might manipulate the results, leading to wrong diagnoses or treatment plans [35]. This could be harmful because it might cause unnecessary treatments or, conversely, result in missing crucial health issues.

6.2.4   Bias and Non-discrimination

Within healthcare, careful attention to gender and sex considerations is essential due to their significant impact on individuals' health and variations in disease patterns [36]. Despite this importance, a substantial number of algorithms utilized in healthcare fail to incorporate these factors and lack mechanisms for detecting bias [37]. Overlooking these critical dimensions in medical algorithms raises significant concerns, as neglecting such considerations is likely to yield suboptimal outcomes and introduce errors, potentially resulting in misdiagnoses and instances of discrimination [18].

Some of these choices are made explicitly by those who design and manufacture these technologies, other choices may be more implicit, for instance, caused by convictions, beliefs, and behavior of those who design new technologies. A typical example is that in the technology sector, there are more male workers than female workers. As a result, women struggling to be in higher-ranked positions are more prone to harassment [38], and technology designs for this environment are more oriented toward males than females. Imbalance in sex and gender representation within medical imaging datasets can also cause biased classifiers for computer-aided diagnosis [39, 40]. Take, for instance, facial recognition tools, which perform better on white, middle-aged men than other categories, because these tools were trained on datasets with white males [10, 41]. Another example is the development and testing of new medicines, which often contain sex biases [42]. In this respect, there is also a growing understanding that, beyond sex, other intersectional differences such as gender and race play an essential role in determining the physical and mental well-being of people, although this is often not thought of in AI development [18, 37].

Some authors highlight that only a multifaceted, more intersectional approach may contribute to addressing the implications of biases in AI for medicine [18]. First and foremost, legal frameworks should evolve to account explicitly for diversity considerations in AI development. Current guidelines often focus on physical safety, overlooking aspects like security, privacy, psychological impacts, and diversity, which are crucial for healthcare applications. Secondly, responsible innovation tools, like the Responsible Research and Innovation (RRI) framework, can guide research processes [43]. Inclusion, anticipation, reflection, responsiveness, and transparency are fundamental principles in the RRI approach, encouraging diverse stakeholder involvement, anticipating adverse consequences, and reflecting on biases from the technology conception, the training datasets, to its implementation [44]. Lastly, a technical approach involves developing discrimination-aware algorithms, using gender-neutral biomarkers, and curating datasets to eliminate biases [45]. The goal is to ensure AI applications are informed, attuned to societal contexts, and respectful of privacy and diversity. This comprehensive strategy seeks to navigate the complexities of AI in medicine, mitigating biases and fostering responsible, inclusive, and diverse research and application.

6.3 Ethical Aspects

This section examines the most relevant ethical aspects such as human dignity, autonomy, and accountability.

6.3.1 Human Dignity

All the basic human rights (e.g., non-discrimination, freedom of expression, freedom of religion, privacy) and core values in ethics (e.g., autonomy, non-maleficence, justice) are to some extent related to dignity. Interference with these values implies interference with human dignity. In other words, dignity is the underlying value or one of the underlying values that needs protection. In ethics, dignity is the clearest way of taking the vulnerabilities of others into account. It focuses on the human condition, which is inherently vulnerable. In human rights law, which focuses on the rights and freedoms of people, human dignity is also the common denominator. The German constitution starts with human dignity (die Würde des Menschen) as the first basic right listed. The same holds for the EU Charter of Fundamental Rights, which opens Article 1 with human dignity. In both legal documents, the right to human dignity is stated to be inviolable; it is an absolute right, meaning that under no circumstances are violations of this right allowed.

Dignity is under pressure in the context of AI [46]. People are increasingly judged upon their digital representation (the digital person) rather than as human beings of flesh and blood [47]. When a person is no longer treated as someone with particular interests, feelings, and commitments, but merely as a bundle of data, her dignity may be compromised. Practices like profiling can reinforce a tendency to regard persons as mere objects [48]. When using AI in radiology, there also exists the risk of focusing on the data rather than the people. This may not always be problematic for research purposes, but it is essential to focus on an individual patient and involve the patient in any decisions for clinical purposes.

AI can also put human dignity under pressure by treating them unfairly. A digital representation of a person can be different from reality in several ways. For instance, the data can be incorrect or incomplete, creating a wrong representation. When using AI in radiology, it is important to be aware of any bias in the datasets and the patterns and knowledge the AI tools produce. In medicine, sex and gender bias is a common problem, which can be perpetuated and even amplified in AI tools [37]. For instance, if drugs were only tested on a male population, their effectiveness and any side effects may be unknown for female patients. In radiology, if the input data is biased toward specific groups of people, the findings may also contain this bias. In this vein, more research is needed to understand what intersectional differences are important to integrate within AI for radiology to ensure these systems are safe to use in different populations.

6.3.2 Autonomy

Autonomy refers to the extent to which people are in control of their lives and the decisions they make. In privacy and data protection, autonomy is closely related to the control people have over their personal data. An important factor in realizing autonomy is properly informing people before making decisions [49]. Consent always boils down to informed consent. However, informing people can be hard in a medical context, in which people may be more vulnerable than usual, may have limited options to choose from, may find it hard to understand medical information, and may experience high levels of stress and anxiety. In radiology, this may be further complicated because of the advanced technologies involved.

Although consent is important, it is a complex mechanism to use. People seem to become increasingly disengaged in consent processes, such that consent decisions fail to have the intended moral effect of giving agency to individuals as autonomous decision-makers [50, 51]. Often, there are (too) many requests for consent [52]. As a result of this, many people unquestioningly accept consent boxes when they resemble other dialog boxes [53]. It would take much time people were to consider every consent request seriously. Moreover, it may often feel as if they have no choice in any case when encountering consent decisions since these are framed as take-it-or-leave-it offers: refusing consent means that a treatment or therapy cannot be started.

When applying AI tools in radiology, properly informing people to ensure their autonomy and autonomous decision-making is even more complicated for other reasons [29]. Typically, AI tools are very complex and opaque. The complexity means that even for experts, it may be hard to understand and explain how the tools work [54]. Furthermore, the continuous improvement of AI tools implies that any explanation is merely a snapshot, as the workings of an AI tool may have further evolved as time passes.

6.3.3 Accountability

The use of AI for law tools can lead to errors in decision-making. If this leads to harm or damages, it raises the question of who is responsible and legally liable. For instance, if an AI prediction tool in radiology overlooks a tumor, a patient may not receive the needed treatment. Or, the other way around, if surgery is performed on the basis of an AI system signaling a concerning tumor, but it turns out there is no tumor at all, harm has been done. In both cases, the question can arise who is liable for this harm.

Typically, errors and bias can occur in all stages of decision-making in which AI is involved. First, the data can contain errors (e.g., the data can be incorrect or incomplete) or can be biased (e.g., by the way the data were collected) [55]. Second, the analysis of the data can be biased, for instance, by the way the data analytics tools are developed and trained. Typically, facial recognition tools perform better on white, middle-aged males than other categories because these tools were trained on datasets with white males [10, 41]. For other people, such as women, people of color, and younger people, the accuracy of the tools decreases. Third, the results that AI tools put forward can be misinterpreted or applied in the wrong way. For instance, if AI tools conclude that a particular group of persons is more likely to commit crimes, this may be a statistically correct conclusion. If, however, based on this profile, law enforcement starts intensive surveillance on this group of people, it may be that they are also putting innocent people under close surveillance (false positives) while at the same time disregarding people that should be focused on (false negatives).

Mistakes and errors can lead to risks, harms, and damages. This raises the question of who is liable for that. It could be the user of the tools. If a radiologist uses an AI tool incorrectly and causes harm, liability is like the wrong use of any other tool [56]. In most jurisdictions, there are also ways to hold (at least to some extent) the owner of the tool liable, which could be the hospital. If it turns out, however, that the AI tool was properly used, but somehow did not function properly, the manufacturer (directly or indirectly via the seller of the tool) of the tool can be liable based on product liability rules.

This is further complicated with the use of AI tools that are self-learning, which complicates the application of any existing liability rules. Typically, an AI tool can make mistakes while still learning the best solution for a problem (similar to how humans sometimes learn on-the-job). Also, AI tools can cause harm while still making optimal decisions. Say, for instance, that an AI tool is used to prioritize patients for surgery. Even with optimal ordering, there may be a patient who has to wait too long to receive surgery and suffers harm from this. The tool is not misused and is not malfunctioning, but it still causes harm. This situation creates a "liability gap," in which liability cannot be allocated in a satisfying way [57, 58]. When applying existing rules for contractual, extra-contractual, or strict liability to AI for law tools yield unsatisfying outcomes, these rules may need to be reconsidered. Additional liability rules could be introduced, but these also create the risk of chilling effects on innovation [59].

6.4   Further Mapping of Legal and Ethical Aspects

Sections 6.2 and 6.3 described the most relevant legal and ethical aspects of the use of AI in radiology. However, this analysis does not provide an exhaustive overview. There may be other relevant aspects to consider, depending on the specific functionalities and applications of an AI system. Several methods are available to map the ethical and legal issues of AI. A typical approach is a data protection impact assessment (DPIA) or simply a privacy impact assessment (PIA) [60]. These methods, mandatory under the GDPR before starting any process or system that collects and processes personal data, help to identify any privacy issues and assess their impact. The results of such an assessment, in turn, can contribute to implementing any (privacy) risk-mitigating measures.

The approach of implementing measures that address privacy issues in the design of technology is called data protection by design (DPbD) or simply privacy by design (PbD) [61, 62]. This is also mandatory under the GDPR. In line with privacy by design, the GDPR also imposes the obligation to consider privacy by default in Article 25 of the GDPR. Privacy by default aims to set defaults in technology in a privacy-friendly mode, for instance, opt-in instead of opt-out. If this approach is taken broader, considering all kinds of values beyond privacy, this approach is called value-sensitive design.

Value-sensitive design (VSD) is a theory that states that important values (like the legal and ethical aspects identified in Sects. 6.2 and 6.3 of this chapter) should be included in the design of new technologies. In other words, those designing and manufacturing new technologies should consider not only functional design requirements, but also legal and ethical design requirements. This theory was developed by Batya Friedman and Peter Kahn at the University of Washington in the late 1980s and early 1990s [63]. As the name of this theory already indicates, it is a design-based approach that tries to implement values into the design of new technologies, as opposed to an application-based approach, in which it tries to address how new technologies are used. As such, VSD must be applied before technologies are produced and put on the market. VSD considers human values throughout the whole process of designing new technologies [64]. It requires that technological teams of designers and engineers are supplemented with other experts, such as experts in ethics, law, and social sciences. The technology experts can establish functionality requirements and the other experts can establish the legal and ethical requirements.

A VSD approach will likely yield technology designed to address legal and ethical issues better. This can be done without loss of functionality and sometimes without extra costs. However, this may not always be the case, as some of these additional requirements may interfere with functionality requirements, which means these must be balanced. Considering legal and ethical design requirements is likely to increase user acceptance and public support for new technologies, which can constitute a long-term interest for companies that develop new technologies.

Although the concept of value-sensitive design sounds interesting, they do not seem to be applied that often in practice. It should be implemented before a new project starts, but it may not seem to be the highest priority in those stages. Also, it can be complicated to develop strategies for value-sensitive design, such as privacy by design, as it requires sophisticated knowledge of the data processing and available approaches to render them more privacy-friendly. And even if experts are working on this, trade-offs between ethical values and business interests may sometimes favor the latter rather than the former. As a result, only limited technological tools exist for implementing value-sensitive design.

6.5   Conclusions

In conclusion, the integration of AI in radiology presents significant opportunities for the field, leveraging the capacity of AI tools to efficiently process vast amounts of medical data and identify patterns imperceptible to human observers. While the focus often centers on technological and medical aspects, this chapter underscores the critical importance of considering legal and ethical dimensions in the development and deployment of AI in radiology. Legal requirements, including those related to safety, privacy, security, and non-discrimination, serve as indispensable safeguards against potential patient harm. Ethical considerations, such as human dignity, autonomy, and accountability, emerge as paramount in navigating the evolving landscape of AI in healthcare.

While acknowledging the limitations of current legal frameworks and ethical norms, this chapter advocated for proactively identifying and qualifying issues, transforming them into design requirements. The exploration of legal aspects emphasizes compliance as a necessity for safeguarding patients. At the same time, ethical scrutiny extends beyond legal obligations, requiring a multifaceted approach to address biases, protect autonomy, and ensure accountability. The comprehensive examination of these legal and ethical facets sets the stage for the development of AI tools in radiology that adhere to regulatory standards and prioritize safety, user-friendliness, and public support.

In the quest for responsible innovation, this chapter introduced methodologies such as impact assessments and value-sensitive design, offering a roadmap to identify, qualify, and address legal and ethical challenges early in the development process. As the integration of AI in radiology continues to advance, adherence to legal and ethical principles emerges not as a hindrance but as a catalyst for fostering innovation that is not only cutting-edge but also conscientious and human-centric.

Acknowledgement E. Fosch-Villaronga is thankful to the Safe and Sound project, a project that has received funding from the European Union's Horizon-ERC program, Grant Agreement No. 101076929.

References

1. Hosny A, Parmar C, Quackenbush J, Schwartz LH, Aerts HJWL. Artificial intelligence in radiology. Nat Rev Cancer. 2018;18:500–10.
2. Arabi H, Zaidi H. Applications of artificial intelligence and deep learning in molecular imaging and radiotherapy. Eur J Hybrid Imaging. 2020;4:17.
3. Custers B, Fosch-Villaronga E. Law and artificial intelligence: regulating ai and applying AI in legal practice. Springer Nature; 2022.
4. Norval C, Janssen H, Cobbe J, Singh J. Data protection and tech startups: the need for attention, support, and scrutiny. Policy Internet. 2021;13:278–99.
5. See the efforts made by the European Commission in light of the General Safety Product Regulation to encourage and honor innovative business initiatives and research that make a difference for consumers via the EU Product Safety Award. https://ec.europa.eu/safety-gate/#/screen/pages/safetyAward
6. Artificial Intelligence Act: deal on comprehensive rules for trustworthy AI. 2023. https://www.europarl.europa.eu/news/en/press-room/20231206 IPR15699/artificial-intelligence-act-deal-on-comprehensive-rules-for-trustworthy-ai
7. Jaremko JL, et al. Canadian association of radiologists white paper on ethical and legal issues related to artificial intelligence in radiology. Can Assoc Radiol J. 2019;70:107–18.

8. D'Antonoli TA. Ethical considerations for artificial intelligence: an overview of the current radiology landscape. Diagn Interv Radiol. 2020;26:504–11.
9. Rustad ML. Products liability for software defects in driverless cars. Rustad Book Proof; 2023.
10. Fosch-Villaronga E, Poulsen A, Søraa RA, Custers B. Gendering algorithms in social media. SIGKDD Explor Newsl. 2021;23:24–31.
11. Daye D, et al. Implementation of clinical artificial intelligence in radiology: who decides and how? Radiology. 2022;305:E62.
12. Geis JR, et al. Ethics of artificial intelligence in radiology: summary of the joint European and North American multisociety statement. Radiology. 2019;293:436–40.
13. Tadavarthi Y, et al. Overview of noninterpretive artificial intelligence models for safety, quality, workflow, and education applications in radiology practice. Radiol Artif Intell. 2022;4:e210114.
14. Ribeiro MT, Singh S, Guestrin C. 'Why should i trust you?': explaining the predictions of any classifier. In: Proceedings of the 22nd ACM SIGKDD International Conference on Knowledge Discovery and Data Mining. New York, NY: Association for Computing Machinery; 2016. p. 1135–44.
15. Winkler JK, et al. Association between surgical skin markings in dermoscopic images and diagnostic performance of a deep learning convolutional neural network for melanoma recognition. JAMA Dermatol. 2019;155:1135–41.
16. Hille EM, Hummel P, Braun M. Meaningful human control over AI for health? A review. J Med Ethics. 2023; https://doi.org/10.1136/jme-2023-109095.
17. Tocchetti A et al. A.I. robustness: a human-centered perspective on technological challenges and opportunities. arXiv [cs.AI]. 2022.
18. Fosch-Villaronga E, Drukarch H, Khanna P, Verhoef T, Custers B. Accounting for diversity in AI for medicine. Comput Law Secur Rep. 2022;47:105735.
19. Pesapane F, Codari M, Sardanelli F. Artificial intelligence in medical imaging: threat or opportunity? Radiologists again at the forefront of innovation in medicine. Eur Radiol Exp. 2018;2:35.
20. Grzybowski A, et al. Correction to: Artificial intelligence for diabetic retinopathy screening: a review. Eye. 2020;34:604.
21. Oakden-Rayner L, Palmer LJ. Artificial intelligence in medicine: validation and study design. In: Ranschaert ER, Morozov S, Algra PR, editors. Artificial intelligence in medical imaging: opportunities, applications and risks. Cham: Springer International Publishing; 2019. p. 83–104.
22. https://digital-strategy.ec.europa.eu/en/library/ethics-guidelines-trustworthy-ai.

23. Nikolinakos NT. EU policy and legal framework for artificial intelligence, robotics and related technologies—the AI Act. Springer Nature; 2023.
24. Radclyffe C, Ribeiro M, Wortham RH. The assessment list for trustworthy artificial intelligence: a review and recommendations. Front Artif Intell. 2023;6:1020592.
25. Mongan J, Kohli M. Artificial intelligence and human life: five lessons for radiology from the 737 MAX disasters. Radiol Artif Intell. 2020;2:e190111.
26. Kelly CJ, Karthikesalingam A, Suleyman M, Corrado G, King D. Key challenges for delivering clinical impact with artificial intelligence. BMC Med. 2019;17:195.
27. Degnan AJ, et al. Perceptual and interpretive error in diagnostic radiology-causes and potential solutions. Acad Radiol. 2019;26:833–45.
28. Bommasani R, et al. On the opportunities and risks of foundation models. arXiv [cs.LG]. 2021.
29. Custers B, Dechesne F, Pieters W, Schermer BW, van der Hof S. Consent and privacy. In: Schaber P, Müller A, editors. Handbook of the ethics of consent. Routledge; 2018. p. 247–58.
30. Amann J, et al. Explainability for artificial intelligence in healthcare: a multidisciplinary perspective. BMC Med Inform Decis Mak. 2020;20:310.
31. Kempt H, Heilinger J-C, Nagel SK. 'I'm afraid I can't let you do that, doctor': meaningful disagreements with AI in medical contexts. AI Soc. 2023;38:1407–14.
32. Mirsky Y, Mahler T, Shelef I, Elovici Y. CT-GAN: malicious tampering of 3D medical imagery using deep learning. USENIX Security Symposium. 2019;461–478.
33. Chu LC, Anandkumar A, Shin HC, Fishman EK. The potential dangers of artificial intelligence for radiology and radiologists. J Am Coll Radiol. 2020;17:1309–11.
34. Ranschaert ER, et al. Advantages, challenges, and risks of artificial intelligence for radiologists. In: Ranschaert ER, Morozov S, Algra PR, editors. Artificial intelligence in medical imaging: opportunities, applications and risks. Cham: Springer International Publishing; 2019. p. 329–46.
35. Yaacoub J-PA, et al. Securing internet of medical things systems: limitations, issues and recommendations. Futur Gener Comput Syst. 2020;105:581–606.
36. Goisauf M, Cano Abadía M. Ethics of AI in radiology: a review of ethical and societal implications. Front Big Data. 2022;5:850383.
37. Cirillo D, et al. Sex and gender differences and biases in artificial intelligence for biomedicine and healthcare. NPJ Digit Med. 2020;3:81.
38. Fichera G, Busch IM, Rimondini M, Motta R, Giraudo C. Is empowerment of female radiologists still needed? Findings of a systematic review. Int J Environ Res Public Health. 2021;18:1542.

39. Larrazabal AJ, Nieto N, Peterson V, Milone DH, Ferrante E. Gender imbalance in medical imaging datasets produces biased classifiers for computer-aided diagnosis. Proc Natl Acad Sci USA. 2020;117:12592–4.
40. Custers BHM. Big Data in wetenschappelijk onderzoek. Justitiële verkenn. 2016;42:8–21.
41. Klare BF, Burge MJ, Klontz JC, Vorder Bruegge RW, Jain AK. Face recognition performance: role of demographic information. IEEE Trans Inf Forensics Secur. 2012;7:1789–801.
42. Merone L, Tsey K, Russell D, Nagle C. Sex inequalities in medical research: a systematic scoping review of the literature. Womens Health Rep (New Rochelle). 2022;3:49–59.
43. von Schomberg R. A vision of responsible research and innovation. In: Responsible innovation. Chichester: John Wiley & Sons, Ltd.; 2013. p. 51–74.
44. Verhoef T, Fosch-Villaronga E. Towards affective computing that works for everyone. arXiv [cs.HC]. 2023.
45. Kamiran F, Calders T, Pechenizkiy M. Techniques for discrimination-free predictive models. In: Custers B, Calders T, Schermer B, Zarsky T, editors. Discrimination and privacy in the information society: data mining and profiling in large databases. Berlin, Heidelberg: Springer; 2013. p. 223–39.
46. Düwell M. Human dignity and the ethics and regulation of technology. Oxford University Press; 2016.
47. Solove, D. J. The future of reputation: gossip, rumor, and privacy on the internet (full text of book). (2007).
48. Bygrave LA. Data protection law: approaching its rationale, logic and limits. Netherlands: Springer; 2002.
49. Custers B, et al. The role of consent in an algorithmic society—its evolution, scope, failings and re-conceptualization. In: Research handbook on EU data protection law. Edward Elgar Publishing; 2022. p. 455–73.
50. Hurd HM. The moral magic of consent. Legal Theory. 1996;2:121–46.
51. Kleinig J. 1 The Nature of Consent. Oxford University Press; 2009.
52. Schermer BW, Custers B, van der Hof S. The crisis of consent: how stronger legal protection may lead to weaker consent in data protection. Ethics Inf Technol. 2014;16:171–82.
53. Böhme R, Köpsell S. Trained to accept? A field experiment on consent dialogs. In: Proceedings of the SIGCHI Conference on Human Factors in Computing Systems 2403–2406. New York, NY: Association for Computing Machinery; 2010.
54. Teeuw, W. et al. Security applications for converging technologies : impact on the constitutional state and the legal order. (2008).
55. Torralba A, Efros AA. Unbiased look at dataset bias. In: CVPR 2011. IEEE; 2011. p. 1521–8.

56. Jorstad KT. Intersection of artificial intelligence and medicine: tort liability in the technological age. J Med Artif Intell. 2020;3:17.
57. De Conca S. Bridging the liability gaps: why ai challenges the existing rules on liability and how to design human-empowering solutions. In: Custers B, Fosch-Villaronga E, editors. Law and artificial intelligence: regulating AI and applying AI in legal practice. The Hague: T.M.C. Asser Press; 2022. p. 239–58.
58. Bertolini A. Robots as products: the case for a realistic analysis of robotic applications and liability rules, vol. 5; 2013. p. 214–47.
59. Büchi M, et al. The chilling effects of algorithmic profiling: mapping the issues. Computer Law & Security Review. 2020;36:105367.
60. Wright D, de Hert P. Privacy impact assessment. Springer; 2012.
61. Cavoukian A. Privacy by design: the definitive workshop. A foreword by Ann Cavoukian, Ph.D. Identity in the Information Society 3. 2010:247–251
62. Custers B, Calders T, Schermer B, Tal Z. Discrimination and privacy in the information society. Berlin, Heidelberg: Springer; 2012.
63. Friedman B, Kahn PH, Borning A, Huldtgren A. Value sensitive design and information systems. In: Doorn N, Schuurbiers D, van de Poel I, Gorman ME, editors. Early engagement and new technologies: opening up the laboratory. Dordrecht: Springer; 2013. p. 55–95.
64. Friedman B, Kahn P, Borning A. Value sensitive design: theory and methods. University of Washington technical report. 2002.

Workflow Integration and Training

7

João Abrantes ⓘ and Willem Grootjans ⓘ

Key Points
- AI integration in radiology improves diagnostic accuracy, efficiency, and patient care through enhanced data management and decision-making processes.
- Successful AI implementation in radiology requires robust informatics networks for secure, swift data transfer and integration into existing healthcare workflows.
- AI technologies enable reallocation of tasks within radiology departments, necessitating new training programs for adapted roles.
- AI applications in radiology can streamline operations from ordering and scheduling to image acquisition, enhancing both workflow and patient outcomes.
- Continuous evaluation and iteration of AI tools in radiology are essential for ensuring long-term effectiveness and sustainability.

J. Abrantes (✉)
Imaging Department, ULSTMAD, Vila Real, Portugal
e-mail: jmvabrantes@chtmad.min-saude.pt

W. Grootjans
Department of Radiology, Leiden University Medical Center, Leiden, Zuid-Holland, The Netherlands
e-mail: w.grootjans@lumc.nl

© The Author(s), under exclusive license to Springer Nature Switzerland AG 2024
E. Ranschaert et al. (eds.), *AI Implementation in Radiology*, Imaging Informatics for Healthcare Professionals,
https://doi.org/10.1007/978-3-031-68942-0_7

7.1   Introduction

The advent of artificial intelligence (AI) in healthcare, particularly within radiology departments, signifies a transformative
shift toward enhanced diagnostic accuracy, efficiency, and patient
care. However, the successful integration of AI technologies into
existing radiological workflows and processes is not without its
challenges. It requires a comprehensive approach that encompasses not only adjustments to workflows but also a strategic
change management plan. This plan must detail the workflow
changes, redefine roles and responsibilities, and ensure that
healthcare professionals are appropriately trained to use and interpret AI outputs effectively.

At the core of any successful AI implementation in radiology,
or the broader healthcare system, lies a robust IT network. This
covers the technical configuration for secure data transfer as well
as the workflow integration of AI tools. It encompasses both hardware, such as servers and network structure, and software for
managing and analyzing data, ensuring that AI results are seamlessly integrated into healthcare processes and decision-making.
For example, an efficient IT network is essential in a radiology
department that uses AI to help identify bone fractures from the
emergency department X-rays. It ensures that X-ray images are
automatically transmitted from the imaging equipment to the AI
software quickly and securely. It also incorporates the AI's results
straight into the Picture Archiving and Communication System
(PACS). This integration makes it possible for medical professionals to make quick, well-informed decisions regarding patient
care by giving them timely access to clinically relevant findings.
In this regard, AI technologies are to be viewed as essential sup-
plements to the vast array of informatics tools and software that
underpin the healthcare system.

The basic workflow of a modern radiology department consists
of several systems, including the electronic health record (EHR),
radiology information system (RIS), and PACS. These systems
are used together and should optimally support the radiology
value chain, as described in Chap. 2. The potential of AI to add
value at each step of the radiology value chain is well recognized.

However, implementation of AI is not without its challenges and a holistic approach to AI implementation should be sought where organizations should structure and align technology, workflows, human resources, and organizational structures to create and sustain value with AI [1].

The adoption of certain AI tools also presents the opportunity, and in some cases the need, for shifting traditional and new tasks and roles to other professionals, who have specific knowledge about the use and management of AI. However, practical implementation of such task differentiation is challenging, because new or adapted para-professionals (e.g., physician assistants or technical physicians) have to be trained, and new workflows consistent with this technology have to be developed. Effective strategies must address the technical, procedural, and human factors involved in this transition as well as a focus on continuous evaluation of performance and developing feedback loops, allowing for iterative improvement and guaranteeing long-term sustainability.

This chapter will explore a variety of both established and emerging applications of AI in the radiological value chain. It will illustrate how AI technologies can streamline departmental operations and exert a significant impact on broader institutional or enterprise-wide processes. Furthermore, the chapter will focus on several aspects of training and retraining professionals for AI adoption, as well as the seamless integration of AI technologies into the radiological workflow.

7.2 Workflow of the Radiology Department

Radiology departments operate a complex workflow. Typically, these departments have digitized substantial parts of the workflow, which are supported by various information systems. The radiology workflow commences with the referral for a radiological examination by a physician, an action typically facilitated through the hospital's EHR. This system is intricately linked with the RIS, ensuring a seamless transition of orders.

Overall, the RIS plays a crucial role in optimizing the operational efficiency of radiology departments, improving the quality of care through better management of patient data, scheduling and reporting, and ensuring accurate financial management. After receiving the examination order, a process of rigorous evaluation and possibly a healthcare insurance pre-authorization is started to confirm the selection of appropriate radiological procedures and protocols. Upon validation, the examination is planned and scheduled by the department's administrative staff.

On the scheduled day, the patient undergoes the radiological procedure. The digitally acquired images are then transmitted to the PACS for secure storage and subsequent analysis. Furthermore, the workflow is supported by an array of clinical front-end software systems, including PACS viewers and advanced visualization packages. These systems provide the possibility to visualize and analyze data by directly querying or receiving image data from the PACS data to support the diagnostic process.

AI technology can enhance the radiological workflow at various stages. The implementation of AI models within the radiological workflow requires the definition of precise rules or triggers for activation. It is crucial to design these triggers to be both unique and timely, guaranteeing that AI-generated results are available at the moment they are needed. This strategic setup ensures that AI tools effectively augment the diagnostic process, providing support where it is most beneficial without disrupting the workflow. The nature of these predefined triggers, such as launching a specific imaging protocol or the arrival of a patient with a particular clinical question, varies based on the department's unique organizational structure and requires thoughtful collaboration between clinicians and IT representatives.

These triggers can be programmed to recognize specific elements in DICOM metadata, such as the name of an imaging protocol, or to identify particular information, like clinical indications, within HL7 message fields. Once activated, AI models may either pull the required imaging data directly from the PACS, or the PACS might push image data to an AI model for analysis. The AI results are subsequently returned to the PACS and made accessible through clinical front-end software. After reporting, information is sent and made available in the EHR.

We can segment this integrated approach in three primary phases [2, 3]:

1. From order entry to image acquisition: This initial phase encompasses the journey from the entry of radiological examination orders through the EHR to the acquisition of images.
2. Workflow orchestration, analysis, prioritization and reporting: This phase involves the transmission of the acquired imaging data to the PACS/VNA, the orchestration of imaging data, the use of AI for advanced analysis and prioritization, and the subsequent evaluation of the acquired imaging data and AI-generated results by the radiologist for interpretation and drafting the final report.
3. Monitoring and business logic: Phase related to the integration of reports and results into the EHR, allowing for ongoing monitoring of workflow efficiencies throughout the entire department using business analytics to optimize operational aspects. It is deeply connected with governance and research efforts to provide continuous improvement and innovation in radiology practices.

7.2.1   From Order Entry to Image Acquisition

7.2.1.1 Ordering of Radiology Examinations

For many departments, optimizing the radiology examination ordering process can yield significant improvements in efficiency and quality. This is particularly important because this process is susceptible to errors and variability. In some cases, up to 26% of ordered radiology examinations fail to meet eligibility criteria, resulting in wasted resources and unnecessary risks to patients [4, 5]. In this context, clinical decision support systems (CDS) have proven to be invaluable, significantly enhancing the process by eliminating erroneous or redundant orders. The incorporation of AI into these systems can further augment their ability to improve task quality and efficiency. Through the real-time, automated extraction and interpretation of clinical data, it becomes feasible to maintain an updated and integrated list of patient issues. Additionally, a system-wide EHR monitoring tool can automatically pinpoint high-value imaging opportunities across a hospital or healthcare system, thereby enhancing the overall quality and efficiency of care delivery. While commercially available solutions are still emerging, several in-house developed tools have been crafted to tackle these challenges. Successfully integrating such tools into the existing workflow requires robust and effective communication among the multiple data sources within a hospital's infrastructure.

7.2.1.2 Scheduling and Screening

The efficiency of scheduling radiology examinations has administrative and operational challenges. Accurate scheduling requires specific medical knowledge, which creates interruptions for both the administrative staff and the radiologists or radiographers they have to consult during the scheduling process. Efficiency is further decreased by the lack of automation of the process of screening for contraindications, which is crucial to patient safety. The complex tasks associated with scheduling and screening can be significantly enhanced with the use of AI models to analyze complex clinical data and identify contraindications to increase administrative efficiency and greater safety [6]. Alert systems can also provide quality control for the evaluation of follow-up exams, such as alerting when a recommended study was not scheduled or the presence of poorly-timed (e.g., prematurely booked) follow-up exams [7]. In addition, AI may evaluate patients' earlier exams for specific findings, such as the presence of pacemakers that would have an impact on MRI exams, expediting both scheduling and screening processes while maintaining patient safety [8].

7.2.1.3 Selection of Imaging Procedures

Selecting the appropriate imaging procedures and protocols is an essential yet time-intensive task in radiology, often requiring significant effort from radiologists and radiographers. While crucial, the requirement of significant resources can lead to delays in patient care. The advent of AI offers the possibility to streamline this process. Initial efforts used traditional machine learning methods, which, despite their effectiveness, required extensive domain-specific expertise for manual feature selection. This reliance on expert knowledge for feature selection posed limitations, as model performance was directly tied to the quality of the selected features.

Recent advancements have shifted focus toward convolutional neural networks (CNNs), which inherently possess the capability to automatically identify predictive features relevant to the task. This shift is exemplified in a study exploring the use of deep neural networks for the selection of CT and MR imaging protocols [9]. In this case, the process is divided into two distinct steps: (1) automated protocol suggestion, which operates without the need for direct supervision by a radiologist (though supervision by a radiographer remains necessary) and (2) the employment of a CDS tool that presents the top three protocol class predictions for final review and confirmation by a radiologist. In instances where the model's predictions exceeded a high confidence threshold (confidence >0.9) and were supported by sufficient training data (over 100 examples), automated protocol selection (mode 1) was implemented with a remarkable 95% accuracy rate. For the remaining cases, which involved a degree of uncertainty (31%), the system defaulted to the CDS (mode 2), requiring manual review, yet still achieving a 92% accuracy rate.

The implementation of semi-automatic or fully automatic protocol selection mechanisms significantly enhances scheduling efficiency, liberating radiologists to focus on more critical diagnostic tasks. This methodology enables the automatic protocoling of the majority of scans, relegating manual review to more complex cases. Furthermore, this streamlined approach has the potential to facilitate direct patient booking, thereby increasing operational efficiency and improving patient throughput in radiology departments.

7.2.1.4 Image Acquisition

In addition to ordering radiological examinations and appropriate protocol selection, AI has an important role during the different steps of image acquisition. An increasing number of imaging equipment manufacturers are integrating AI-assisted technologies directly into their devices. These AI models assist radiographers in patient positioning and optimize radiation dose delivered to the patient (in case of CT imaging), ensuring the capture of consistent, high-quality images. Such direct integration within the scanner's software streamlines workflow, reduces the need for manual adjustments, and minimizes the risk of repeat exams due to positioning errors. Presently, modern CT, MR, and PET scanners are equipped with these functionalities and are commercially available. Such functionalities are also available for conventional X-rays, where AI-enhanced positioning systems aid in precise patient placement [7]. Additionally, a number of manufacturers provide a separate real-time feedback system on X-ray machines that informs radiographers about image quality and necessity of retakes, which is invaluable for complex examinations where optimal positioning is crucial.

AI also enhances the capability of selecting optimal imaging protocols based on previous imaging exams, enabling precise comparisons of technical parameters like contrast-enhanced phases on CT, which are beneficial for subsequent MRI assessments. This facilitates consistent imaging across time frames and modalities, vital for tracking disease progression or assessing treatment efficacy [10].

A significant breakthrough has been in AI-guided image reconstruction, which dramatically improves image quality (e.g., noise reduction). Using these innovations provides the possibility to shorten image acquisition times for MR and PET scans and decreases patient exposure to ionizing radiation in PET and CT [11]. Moreover, AI-reconstructed images allow for substantial reductions in contrast material usage; for instance, MRI brain imaging can achieve a tenfold reduction in gadolinium dose, significantly lowering the risk associated with IV contrast while maintaining sufficient image quality [12]. Furthermore, AI-based motion correction can significantly improve image quality by removing deteriorating motion artifacts from images.

Lastly, the advent of AI models capable of creating synthetic datasets marks an important class of models in radiological imaging. These generative AI models can create new imaging data (e.g., new imaging series or simulated images from a different modality). Some examples are models that transform MR images into synthetic CT scans or generate virtual contrast-enhanced CT images from non-contrast scans [13, 14]. These models can reduce the number of required radiological examinations, amount of required contrast material, or exposure to ionizing radiation. While many of these AI tools are integrated into scanner software, vendor-neutral platforms also exist, enabling broader application across different systems and devices. This spectrum of AI applications not only improves diagnostic accuracy and patient safety but also paves the way for more efficient and patient-centric radiology practices (Box 7.1).

Box 7.1: Insight from Practice: AI-Enhanced MRI Quality and Efficiency
The adoption of AI-based deep learning reconstructions in MRI equipment at a large private hospital in Portugal has led to remarkable improvements:

- **Image quality boost:** With the ability to produce images almost on par with 3 tesla units, 1.5 tesla MRI equipment are now more often used for detailed tests such as hip and prostate exams as well as high-resolution neuroimaging (pituitary, orbits).
- **Reduction of acquisition time:** This innovation has significantly reduced MRI wait times, improving patient scheduling effectiveness, providing a time buffer between scheduled exams.
- **Preference of radiologists:** The superior results have led some radiologists to preferentially choose to report exams from AI-enhanced machines, providing great feedback on the impact of this technology.

7.2.2 Workflow Orchestration, Analysis, Prioritization and Reporting

7.2.2.1 Application for Workflow Orchestration and Work Distribution

Seamless integration of AI into radiological workflows hinges on the efficient routing of information and imaging data. However, programming such forwarding rules often results in a rigid workflow with limited adaptability. For instance, any alteration in protocol names due to new insights or organizational changes requires corresponding adjustments in related processes and workflow triggers. As the number of AI applications grows and workflow complexity increases, these inflexible mechanisms heighten the risk of workflow disruptions, such as incorrect or incomplete data forwarding or failure to activate AI applications.

A promising solution lies in leveraging AI for pixel-based analysis of acquired examinations, allowing for the automatic identification of image attributes independent of the associated DICOM tags. This approach enables data recognition at the image level (e.g., a contrast-enhanced chest CT) rather than relying solely on metadata, fostering a more resilient workflow. Such pixel-based recognition can streamline that the orchestration of AI applications by ensuring data is directed to the appropriate destinations in a more flexible manner.

Beyond addressing workflow-related challenges, pixel-based recognition can aid radiologists in the reporting phase of examinations. For example, such an approach can automate the selection of hanging protocols to display the intended anatomical region, reconstruction, or sequence. Presently, these hanging protocols typically rely on DICOM metadata, such as imaging protocol names and series descriptions, which introduces similar challenges to those encountered in the automated forwarding of imaging data within the workflow. Optimizing the routing of examinations to the correct subspecialty radiologists, or to those available at the time, could be performed using such pixel-based recognition, which can significantly enhance workflow efficiency. Although radiologists' shifts are traditionally scheduled according to their subspecialties, this method can lead to the misrouting of examinations. The development of tools that provide detailed insights into radiologists' subspecialties and real-time availability promises a dynamic and scalable solution for examination assignment. By circumventing the limitations of fixed scheduling, such advancements could allow for a more flexible and efficient resource allocation, marking a significant step forward in the evolution of radiological practices.

7.2.2.2 Worklist Prioritization

Radiology worklists have historically been arranged based on the provisional diagnosis, with cases being prioritized based on the perceived urgency of the patient's condition. Finding and ranking cases with potentially important findings are made possible by the results that AI applications provide, which provide a means of prioritizing critical findings. In addition to lowering medico-legal risks, morbidity and death rates, this change could additionally decrease the need for clinical staff to interrupt workflows in order to reply to urgent results questions. There are several applications available that are capable of detecting acute findings (e.g., pneumothorax, stroke, fractures, pulmonary embolism, and intracranial hemorrhage) on images. While the detection of acute findings by AI significantly enhances patient safety and the quality of care, its utility in worklist prioritization extends further. AI can provide detailed insights into exam complexity, such as the number of lung nodules identified in a chest CT scan, and the severity of detected abnormalities (Box 7.2). This advanced worklist management, enabled by AI, proves invaluable in networks spanning multiple hospitals by facilitating a strategic redistribution of cases. It allows for the allocation of exams based on various factors, including the clinical experience, subspecialty, and current workload of radiologists. Moreover, AI prioritization can expedite the referral process for patients in need of complex or specialized care, potentially available only at specific hospitals or care centers.

The impact of AI in enhancing worklist prioritization is particularly marked in clinical settings burdened by high case volumes and extended turnaround times. In environments where operational efficiency is already optimized, the incremental benefits of AI-driven prioritization may be less pronounced. However, when implementing AI for worklist prioritization, it is crucial to consider any potential downsides. A significant challenge is the complexity introduced by employing various prioritization tools for different body parts across diverse examinations. Addressing this issue demands strategic decisions about the hierarchy of exam priorities. Leveraging the EHR to incorporate the patient's clinical context offers a solution, enabling a more informed and nuanced approach to prioritization.

Box 7.2: Insight from Practice: AI-Enhanced Worklists
Providing information on factors such as exam complexity, and distinguishing between incidental and non-incidental findings in the PACS before the radiologist begins the exam has been shown to benefit clinical practice:

- **Radiologists know what to expect:** Tackling more complex and challenging exams early on, when the clinician is in a "high energy" state, allows for thorough evaluation. This approach ensures the necessary focus is given to provide clinically impactful results.
- **Balancing workload:** Using information on expected exam complexity helps balance the workload among radiologists, ensuring everyone receives a fair share of both straightforward and challenging cases.

7.2.2.3 Reporting

Many AI applications focus on the reporting phase of the radiology workflow. Activities during the reporting phase of the workflow that can be enhanced with AI results include detection and quantification of findings in images, or applications that assist with the reporting process itself. Traditionally, much effort focused on the creation of computer-assisted diagnosis (CAD) applications that had the capability to automatically detect and mark findings in images. Developments in AI technology, particularly deep learning algorithms, resulted in the development of applications that have high sensitivity for detection of pathologies and have shown to assist radiologists in reading images. Many of these applications also provide the possibility to measure and quantify these findings, such as measurements of target lesions in oncological assessments or volume change over time that are relevant for treatment monitoring. Although these applications can provide significant assistance in the reporting phase, seamless integration of AI results in the report is key to provide the anticipated benefits. Furthermore, a dynamic interaction between the end user and AI-result is key, where it is still possible to adjust a lesion contour based on expert input. Although there is much focus on such dynamic interactions, there are still no standard integrations and the possibility to dynamically interact with AI results will depend on the vendor of the AI application and clinical front-end software.

Using natural language processing (NLP) can also bring value to the radiology reporting workflow. NLP tasks, such as summarizing previous exams, generating exam impressions, and identifying findings that require follow-up, are use cases that can streamline the reporting process. It can also improve report quality by alerting radiologists to potential errors, such as incorrect side references or omitted key findings mentioned in previous reports. Production of contextual reports that are suited to particular illnesses, clinical indications and end users, or the capacity of AI to translate reports into multiple languages can also enhance the clinical impact of radiological exams. The use of large language models has brought remarkable improvements in these areas, outperforming traditional NLP methods in the ability to process complex medical language. In Chap. 9 ("The impact of AI on radiology reporting"), more information on AI-based structured reporting can be found.

7.2.3 Monitoring and Business Logic

7.2.3.1 Coding and Billing

The use of computer-assisted coding, which uses a rules engine to identify proposed medical codes from clinical records, has resulted in a 30% increase in clinical coding productivity. Though useful, it is not totally automated since coders must review every recommended code, and it only works with structured data, despite the fact that analytics reveal that the majority of EHR data (80%) is unstructured [15]. Natural language processing can be used to automate the assignment of billing codes, significantly reducing manual errors and speeding up the billing process. In cases with higher confidence levels, the codes are transmitted directly to billing. The industry standard for autonomous coding is achieving 95% accuracy and when fully optimized, autonomous coding can complete radiology coding workflows within seconds, making cases available for billing up to 3 days sooner [15].

By analyzing billing data to identify discrepancies or unusual patterns, AI can also be of use for regulatory compliance and fraud detection, ensuring adherence to healthcare standards and minimizing legal risks.

7.3   Integration Plan

After establishing a plan for which AI applications to adopt, medical institutions can determine an integration plan for the required applications. Medical institutions have to decide to which extent AI applications will be hosted on-premise or if there is a possibility to host them in the cloud. Additionally, they may choose single-point solutions or a diverse range of applications that interact at various stages in the radiological workflow. Such an integration plan covers a wide array of components. It includes data sharing and routing, and the incorporation of AI results into clinical front-end software such as PACS, advanced viewers, or EHRs. The plan also addresses task prioritization and curation, which involves users interacting with AI results to verify and adjust them as necessary. Additionally, it encompasses the monitoring of AI applications, along with providing resources for their support and maintenance.

7.3.1 On-Premise or Cloud Service

While AI applications can operate entirely on premises within the medical institution's firewall, there is an increasing trend to host such applications using cloud-based services. This means that the hosting of AI applications, as well as the processing of medical data, takes place outside the firewall of the medical institution. Using cloud services for AI analysis offers specific advantages. The first advantage is that the hardware requirements for a medical institution will significantly decrease as the necessary computational capacity is provided by the cloud service. The second advantage is that the responsibility for updating and reconfiguring AI applications will be centralized in the cloud service and performed by the platform provider. Consequently, medical institutions will automatically run the latest version of the AI application available on the cloud service, eliminating the need to continuously allocate resources for updating a diverse range of AI applications. With a cloud-based solution, data from the hospital will be transferred through secure connections to the cloud service hosting the AI applications. The appropriate de-identification and re-identification of data will occur within the medical institution's firewalls using an on-premise installed gateway. However, it is essential to note that in a number of countries, the use of cloud services is either prohibited by legislation or only available to a limited extent. In such instances, hosting AI by means of on-premise solutions might be the only viable option for that particular institution. Furthermore, not all commercially available AI solutions currently support cloud-based implementations. Therefore, the choice for on-premise or cloud solution should be carefully evaluated by the medical institution.

7.3.2 Single-Point Implementations or AI Platform?

If a limited number of AI applications are expected to sufficiently optimize the clinical workflow, medical institutions can opt for a strategy to host these applications using on-premise virtual machines (VMs). The advantage of local VM hosting is that implementations are more straightforward and data will remain within the institution's firewall at all times. However, as the demand for implementing more AI applications grows, integrating AI technology through a vendor-neutral AI (VNAI) platform is expected to be more beneficial for institutions that need multiple AI applications to obtain the required benefits of AI-enhanced workflows. The reason for this is that scaling the number of AI applications using separate VMs becomes demanding and challenging to maintain. The use of multiple VMs can increase complexity and elevate the probability of downtime or failures, due to interactions among diverse software systems. Managing multiple VMs requires careful orchestration and coordination, as each virtualized instance operates as an independent system within the overall infrastructure. Complexity increases due to the need for effective communication and synchronization between different VMs. Configuring, maintaining, and troubleshooting multiple VMs can be challenging, where potential misconfigurations, conflicts, or compatibility issues between software systems can lead to operational disruptions and downtime. Additionally, the use of available hardware is typically more inefficient, as VMs are not always active and can spend a considerable amount of time idling.

In contrast, VNAI platforms can host a variety of AI applications in a standardized fashion, usually by means of containerized implementations. The use of Docker containers simplifies the deployment, scaling, and management of AI applications in radiology by packaging them into separate containers. This ensures that applications run consistently across different computing environments, provide isolation from other applications, and support scalability. Consequently, it facilitates the rapid deployment and updating of AI models, thereby improving operational reliability in radiological practices. In addition to hosting a large variety of AI applications, an AI platform typically has a workflow orchestrator or workflow engine, responsible for the centralized routing of data and information. Furthermore, the advantage of a VNAI platform is that available hardware can be dynamically allocated to specific AI applications as needed. Lastly, the use of a VNA should enable quicker testing of available AI applications, as it falls under a broader umbrella data processing agreement (DPA), eliminating the need to sign individual DPAs with many different vendors.

7.4 Seamless Integration in the Radiology Workflow

Upon selecting a suitable AI integration plan for the medical institution and acquiring the initial AI applications, the integration of AI into the workflow can commence. When considering the integration of AI applications in the radiological workflow, it is important to realize that most AI applications are headless, meaning that they have no typical graphical user interface (GUI) to interact with. In order to successfully integrate a headless application into a clinical workflow, it requires an input and a designated destination for storing output (the AI results). The input for the AI application will come from systems that act as a data source. In case of imaging data, this can be a database on the modality itself or more commonly the PACS. For clinical data, the data source is typically the EHR and/or derivative databases derived from the EHR.

7.4.1 Integration

To achieve a seamless integration, the AI application is connected to a data source and rules are established to facilitate automated transfer of data to the AI application. The criteria used to select and forward data can be based on specific information within

DICOM data, such as information stored in specific DICOM tags or HL7 messages. However, formulating rules for data forwarding is not always straightforward and depends on the required level of specificity. If the criteria for data selection need to be highly specific, the filtering criteria will be narrow, potentially leading to the exclusion of some data from automatic forwarding. Conversely, using criteria that are too broad may result in excessive data being forwarded to the AI application, leading to increased network bandwidth costs, queuing, and subsequent delays in data processing. To ensure precise data selection for current and future AI applications, medical institutions might have to consider adjusting existing protocol names or adding specific tags to data. Additionally, and as previously stated in Sect. 7.2.2 (DICOM routing and AI orchestrating), pixel-based AI models can further enhance this logic, using image data to correctly orchestrate exams, independent of DICOM metadata or information contained in HL7 messages. This refinement aims to improve data selection accuracy, making it better suited for evolving AI technologies.

7.4.2 Interacting with AI

Seamless integration involves more than just technical implementation of AI. Another important aspect to take into consideration is the experience of the end user, making sure that AI results can, if necessary, be corrected with minimal effort and will not cause any significant disruptions. In this regard, end user interaction and ergonomics (e.g., number of mouse clicks) are important measures to take into consideration. Before this can be achieved, it is important to realize that the output of AI applications has to be stored in appropriate databases to be accessed by software applications with which users can interact. These software applications are GUI-equipped and permit the user to interact, review, or modify the AI results. Software systems with such an interface are typically used in routine clinical workflows, such as the PACS viewer or advanced visualization software. In a number of cases, the AI vendor supplies proprietary software with a GUI for interacting with the AI results. Consequently, the output of the AI application needs to be examined and modified using this proprietary software as an intermediary step. After reviewing the AI results using AI vendor-specific software, the AI results are typically archived in the PACS. Although such an integration where multiple GUI-equipped software interfaces are involved is possible, general consensus among clinical end users is that the number of software applications should be limited to maintain a smooth workflow. This is particularly the case when the number of AI applications increases. Therefore, integration of AI results in clinical front-end systems is an important requirement. Most commercially available AI applications have to some degree a possibility to send output to the PACS, where radiologists are able to view the results in the PACS viewer. Therefore, the output files generated by AI applications typically adhere to DICOM standards, which can, for example, be DICOM structured reporting (SR) objects or DICOM encapsulated PDFs. This conformity provides the flexibility to integrate AI-generated results into a variety of clinically available software applications. Although different file types have been used for exporting AI-generated results, the most common formats include encapsulated documents (e.g., PDF files containing result reports), annotations, and measurements (graphical overlays, text annotations), or structured reports.

7.5   Training of Professionals

In addition to seamless integration in clinical workflows, successful implementation and use of AI applications strongly depend upon the thorough training and familiarization of users with these new technologies. This process is critical not only for leveraging AI's full potential but also for mitigating the risks associated with its adoption, including cognitive biases such as automation bias or automation neglect, and other forms of bias that may arise with prolonged use. Training of radiology practitioners such as radiologists and radiographers in AI can be done in several ways and should be an integral and ongoing part of the department strategy when implementing AI applications into clinical practice. By adopting a structured approach to user training, users can be actively engaged with new AI technology, allowing them to form their own understanding of AI tools by interacting with them directly. This could be done by means of hands-on workshops, simulation exercises, and problem-based learning scenarios where professionals apply AI technology to real-world cases, thereby contextualizing their learning and enhancing its relevance to their daily work.

Practical learning is an important factor that will help radiologists, radiographers, and other radiology practitioners in understanding AI-enhanced workflows. Practical learning scenarios help in showing the use of AI applications in combination with their intricate and highly specialized nature of their work. The complexity of interpreting medical images, understanding anatomical variations, and applying this knowledge to diagnose and treat patients demands a hands-on approach to learning. Engaging directly with AI tools through practice allows these professionals to develop the nuanced skills and intuitive judgment necessary for making decisions in a clinical setting and reinforces theoretical knowledge.

7.5.1 The AI Learning Lab

Considering the challenges associated with selecting suitable AI applications and providing practical training simultaneously, having a dynamic learning and testing environment where new AI applications can be explored, tested, and evaluated can significantly facilitate adoption and acceptance by end users. Having such an environment, or AI learning lab, makes it possible to set up pilot and validation experiments that can assist in selecting high potential applications beforehand. This is of particular importance considering that vendors may offer similar AI solutions for specific radiological tasks, where selecting the best available solution is challenging. Having prior knowledge on the performance and acceptance of particular AI applications by end users mitigates the risk of investing excessive time in testing and integrating multiple applications in clinical operations without reaching the expected benefits.

There are different possibilities to host an AI learning lab, where an institution can opt for a completely online virtual environment or create a real physical workspace with one or more radiological workstations. Having a physical space has the advantage of bringing multiple stakeholders together and providing experiments with AI that simulate clinical practice as closely as possible. This setup allows practitioners to evaluate these cases both with and without AI-assisted results, providing a hands-on experience of AI technology in action. Such direct engagement enables practitioners to understand the practical implications of AI, from improving diagnostic accuracy to streamlining workflow processes. By simulating real-world conditions, the AI learning lab serves as an invaluable tool for bridging the gap between theoretical knowledge and practical application, fostering a deeper appreciation, and understanding of how AI can be integrated into radiological practice to enhance patient care.

The concept of task differentiation, where the domain and responsibilities of professions shift, is supported by the use of such an AI learning lab. The learning lab in this setting could provide a comprehensive training programme for professions to ensure that practitioners are proficient in performing new tasks with AI support. This includes not just technical skills, but also the ability to interpret AI-generated insights and understanding capabilities and limitations within the clinical context. Therefore, an AI learning lab should not only focus on a single profession but encompass the entire spectrum of potential end users that can interact with AI applications. Tailored training modules within the AI learning lab can address the unique roles and contributions of radiologists, radiographers, and radiology assistants, ensuring each group acquires the specific skills and knowledge needed to thrive in an AI-enhanced workflow. This approach supports the creation of a collaborative environment where every professional can contribute to the optimization of patient care. Finally, the AI learning lab can be used to establish a feedback mechanism to continuously assess the effectiveness of task differentiation and performance of practitioners, allowing for adjustments as needed to ensure high-quality patient care.

7.6 Conclusions

In this chapter, several requirements and strategic considerations essential for the successful adoption of AI within radiology workflows were discussed. The deployment and effective use of AI can significantly refine the diagnostic process, enrich radiological reports, and optimize workflow efficiency through advanced data analysis and automated systems. Central to the integration of AI applications is their seamless integration into existing IT networks, enabling automated data transfer between different applications and ensuring timely availability of results. This involves setting precise activation triggers for AI applications to ensure their effectiveness at critical points in the workflow, thereby enhancing decision-making processes without disrupting standard operational protocols. Such strategic implementations underscore the necessity for a dynamic and adaptable integration plan that addresses both the technical and human elements of radiology practices.

Additionally, the implementation of AI in radiology requires a multidisciplinary approach involving detailed planning, the redefinition of professional roles, and extensive training of healthcare personnel. Proper education and familiarization with AI technologies empower radiologists and other medical staff to fully utilize these tools, ensuring they complement rather than complicate the diagnostic process. The concept of an AI learning lab is invaluable in this context. Such a facility offers a hands-on environment where professionals can engage with AI technologies under controlled conditions, simulating real-world scenarios. This highlights that enhancing radiology workflows with AI technology extends beyond technological upgrades, requiring adjustments in workflow management, stakeholder engagement, and continuous performance evaluation to ensure sustainable integration.

References

1. Kim B, Romeijn S, Van Buchem M, Mehrizi MHR, Grootjans W. A holistic approach to implementing artificial intelligence in radiology. Insights Imaging. 2024;15:22. https://doi.org/10.1186/s13244-023-01586-4.
2. Kotter E. Basic workflow of medical imaging. In: Van Ooijen PMA, editor. Basic knowledge of medical imaging informatics. Cham: Springer International Publishing; 2021. p. 41–53.
3. Wiggins WF, Magudia K, Schmidt TMS, O'Connor SD, Carr CD, Kohli MD, Andriole KP. Imaging AI in practice: a demonstration of future workflow using integration standards. Radiol Artif Intell. 2021;3:e210152. https://doi.org/10.1148/ryai.2021210152.
4. Lehnert BE, Bree RL. Analysis of appropriateness of outpatient CT and MRI referred from primary care clinics at an academic medical center: how critical is the need for improved decision support? J Am Coll Radiol. 2010;7:192–7. https://doi.org/10.1016/j.jacr.2009.11.010.
5. Pierre K, Haneberg AG, Kwak S, Peters KR, Hochhegger B, Sananmuang T, Tunlayadechanont P, Tighe PJ, Mancuso A, Forghani R. Applications of artificial intelligence in the radiology roundtrip: process streamlining, workflow optimization, and beyond. Semin Roentgenol. 2023;58:158–69. https://doi.org/10.1053/j.ro.2023.02.003.
6. Bizzo BC, Almeida RR, Michalski MH, Alkasab TK. Artificial intelligence and clinical decision support for radiologists and referring providers. J Am Coll Radiol. 2019;16:1351–6. https://doi.org/10.1016/j.jacr.2019.06.010.
7. Letourneau-Guillon L, Camirand D, Guilbert F, Forghani R. Artificial intelligence applications for workflow, process optimization and predictive analytics. Neuroimaging Clin N Am. 2020;30:e1–e15. https://doi.org/10.1016/j.nic.2020.08.008.
8. Thurston MDV, Kim DH, Wit HK. Neural network detection of pacemakers for MRI safety. J Digit Imaging. 2022;35:1673–80. https://doi.org/10.1007/s10278-022-00663-2.
9. Kalra A, Chakraborty A, Fine B, Reicher J. Machine learning for automation of radiology protocols for quality and efficiency improvement. J Am College Radiol. 2020;17:1149–58. https://doi.org/10.1016/j.jacr.2020.03.012.
10. Choy G, Khalilzadeh O, Michalski M, Do S, Samir AE, Pianykh OS, Geis JR, Pandharipande PV, Brink JA, Dreyer KJ. Current applications and future impact of machine learning in radiology. Radiology. 2018;288:318–28. https://doi.org/10.1148/radiol.2018171820.
11. Zhao T, McNitt-Gray M, Ruan D. A convolutional neural network for ultra-low-dose CT denoising and emphysema screening. Med Phys. 2019;46:3941–50. https://doi.org/10.1002/mp.13666.

12. Gong E, Pauly JM, Wintermark M, Zaharchuk G. Deep learning enables reduced gadolinium dose for contrast-enhanced brain MRI. Magn Reson Imaging. 2018;48:330–40. https://doi.org/10.1002/jmri.25970.
13. Emami H, Dong M, Nejad-Davarani SP, Glide-Hurst CK. Generating synthetic CTs from magnetic resonance images using generative adversarial networks. Med Phys. 2018;45:3627–36. https://doi.org/10.1002/mp.13047.
14. Sanders JW, Chen HS, Johnson JM, Schomer DF, Jimenez JE, Ma J, Liu H. Synthetic generation of DSC-MRI-derived relative CBV maps from DCE MRI of brain tumors. Magn Reson Med. 2021;85:469–79. https://doi.org/10.1002/mrm.28432.
15. DeliverHealth. Autonomous Coding for Radiology 101: Boost accuracy with NLP. 2022. https://deliverhealth.com/blog/autonomous-coding-for-radiology-101-boost-accuracy-with-nlp/.

Evaluation, Monitoring, and Improvement

8

Willem Grootjans

Key Points
- Integration of business intelligence principles is crucial for evaluating AI's impact on radiology.
- Key performance indicators can be used to quantify changes driven by AI.
- Determining the impact of multiple AI solutions demand a robust performance monitoring system.
- With information provided by KPIs, informed decisions can be made to optimise clinical practice.

8.1 Radiology and Business Intelligence

With the recognition of artificial intelligence (AI) as a key technology for advancing and sustaining high-quality future radiological services, an important question arises: how can we effectively measure and validate its impact on day-to-day radiology operations? This question is becoming more relevant given

W. Grootjans (✉)
Department of Radiology, Leiden University Medical Center,
Leiden, Zuid-Holland, The Netherlands
e-mail: w.grootjans@lumc.nl

© The Author(s), under exclusive license to Springer Nature Switzerland AG 2024
E. Ranschaert et al. (eds.), *AI Implementation in Radiology*, Imaging Informatics for Healthcare Professionals,
https://doi.org/10.1007/978-3-031-68942-0_8

the fast paced developments that AI technology is currently going through, with more and more AI applications being introduced to the market [1, 2]. This means that for a particular radiology department or medical institution, it becomes more challenging to create a portfolio with AI technologies that optimally aligns with strategic missions and goals of the organisation. Therefore, in order to evaluate whether AI has the intended impact, it is important to have monitoring systems in place that are capable of tracking key performance aspects that are aligned with the established organisational success criteria and strategic goals. Based on these performance metrics, departments are able to make informed decisions regarding optimisations of daily operations, resource management, cost containment, forecasting, and planning as well as quality improvement. This means that the relevance of incorporating the principles of business intelligence (BI) becomes more and more important for the field of radiology.

The concept of BI is employed across many different organisations and enterprises. It essentially comprises a set of different strategies and technologies for the purpose of analysing data and management of business information [3–5]. At the core of these technologies and strategies lies the use of data that offer insights into how the organisation functions. This data can be categorised as being internal, meaning that data is sourced from within the organisation, or external, where data is derived from sources outside the organisational boundaries. It is usually the combination of different internal and external data sources that provide a complete picture that can be used by the organisation to make well-informed policy decisions. In the context of radiology, BI involves the monitoring of performance metrics that enable the identification of potential bottlenecks, inefficiencies, and opportunities for optimisation of radiological workflows and processes. However, with many different software systems and data sources, setting up an effective BI operation in a radiology department is complex. It is an ongoing process that requires collaboration between different stakeholders, adaptability, and a commitment to leveraging data for continuous improvement in patient care and operational efficiency. Furthermore, the current landscape of AI technology, characterised by narrow applications with a diverse set of requirements for implementation, introduces additional layers of complexity to a BI system [6]. Nevertheless, as the role of AI technology continues to grow, there is a pressing need to incorporate BI for regular assessment of the impact of AI technology on radiological operations. This involves compiling a portfolio of applications specific for the medical institution that effectively supports and optimises these operations. This chapter will offer an introduction to the use of BI in radiology, with a focus on AI technology. The specific requirements for such a system will be discussed and concepts on effectively utilising BI for optimising radiological workflows with AI will be explored.

8.2 Aligning with the Organisation

Before an effective BI framework can be established, it is important to establish success criteria for the radiology department. Success criteria for a radiology department can vary and should align with the broader organisational goals of the healthcare institution. Eventually, it is these institutional goals that serve as the foundation for the strategic direction of the entire medical organisation, encompassing areas such as patient care, operational efficiency, and financial sustainability [7] By closely aligning the success criteria of the radiology department with these broader organisational objectives, a cohesive and synergistic approach can be achieved, facilitating not only the achievement of departmental goals but also contributing to the overall success of the healthcare institution. By having a clear view on the organisational goals, the department can identify and prioritise specific points in the radiological operations that can be improved as well as anticipate expected changes in the near future [7]. This can, for example, be related to optimising specific workflows, enhancing resource utilisation, improving quality of care, monitoring performance metrics, supporting strategic decision-making, ensuring regulatory compliance, and facilitating research and education initiatives. When aligning with institutional goals, it is important to engage with stakeholders such as institutional management and different departments in order to formulate and effectively communicate the goals of the radiology department.

Furthermore, incorporating benchmarking into the strategic planning process is essential for setting realistic and achievable goals and objectives for both the institution and radiology department. By evaluating how similar departments at other institutions perform, benchmarking provides valuable insights into best practices, innovative strategies, and performance standards. [8] This comparative analysis helps to ensure that the goals and objectives formulated for the radiology department are not only aligned with the broader organisational goals but are also competitive and reflective of industry standards. As such, benchmarking should be an integral part of the initial planning phase, enabling the department to identify areas where it can excel or needs improvement. This assessment should consider various factors, including patient outcomes, operational efficiencies, technological advancements, and financial performance, among others. By integrating benchmarking data, the radiology department can more accurately define its success criteria, ensuring they are both aspirational and grounded in the reality of the current radiological landscape. This strategic approach facilitates a more targeted and effective path toward enhancing patient-centric care, leveraging AI technologies, and achieving overall excellence in radiological services. Benchmarking thus acts as a critical tool in refining the strategic direction of the radiology department, ensuring that its goals and objectives are not only ambitious but also attainable and relevant to the evolving demands of healthcare delivery.

With the departmental goals established, it is important to define specific objectives that will support the department in successfully achieving these goals. Although goals and objectives are often used interchangeably, they are not similar. Goals typically define success by specifying desired outcomes or end results, providing a general direction for the organisation. An objective, on the other hand, is a specific, measurable, time-bound target that serves as a step toward achieving a broader goal. Thus objectives are more concrete and provide a clear focus for actions and efforts. Goals and objectives therefore vary with respect to scope (broad versus narrow), measurability (qualitative versus quantitative), and timeframe (long-term versus short-term). Furthermore, there is a hierarchical difference, where an objective is always in service of a goal. For example, an institutional goal might be to enhance patient-centric care across healthcare services. The accompanying goal of the radiology department could be as follows: incorporate AI technologies to enhance diagnostic precision and workflow efficiency in radiological imaging services. Subsequently, objectives can be formulated that support these goals: (1) Implement AI applications within the next 6 months to expedite diagnosis and improve accuracy rates by 15%, (2) implement AI-assisted patient triage systems within the next year to prioritise and fast-track critical cases and reduce turnaround time by 20%, (3) establish continuous training programs for radiology staff on the use of AI and ensure that at least 95% of the staff obtains proficiency certificates and use AI in clinical practice.

Furthermore, a clear formulation of both goals and objectives is of importance to make sure to know when they have been reached. In this regard, goals and objectives should be specific, measurable, achievable, relevant, and time-bound (SMART) [9]. Formulating objectives and goals according to the SMART criteria ensures the definition of relevant performance metrics to track progress toward specific goals and objectives. Having specific goals and objectives formulated, the cycle of monitoring progress begins with data collection, followed by analysis and presentation of performance metrics in appropriate dashboards. Departments can then make informed decisions based on the current situation, identifying potential issues and taking action to address them effectively. Figure 8.1 depicts the cycle of monitoring and steering of processes through the use of performance metrics. It is important to realise that goals and objectives are not always static, but can be subjected to changes over time, particularly in an evolving technological and healthcare landscape. Regular evaluation and adjustment of these criteria based on performance assessments and feedback are essential for continuous improvement.

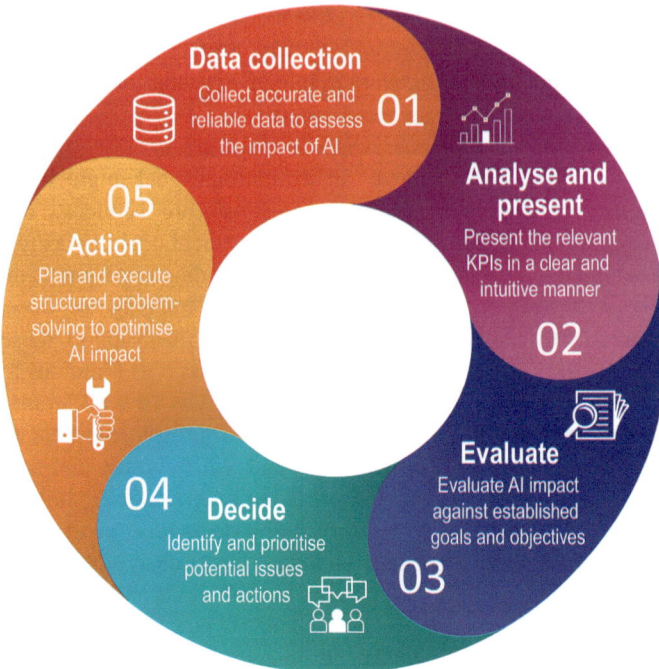

Fig. 8.1 Different steps in monitoring the impact of artificial intelligence (AI) technology on radiology operations. Based on the collection and analysis of relevant data, specific performance metrics such as key performance indicators (KPIs) can be measured. Using the KPI data, department management can identify and prioritise issues, and subsequently take action through structured problem-solving approaches. Subsequent review of the outcomes of improvement initiatives allows for informed decisions—whether to maintain the implementation, make adjustments, or, in the ultimate case, conclude that the proposed solution is not yielding satisfactory results and requires re-evaluation

8.3   Data Collection

8.3.1   Data Warehouse

A key component of BI in radiology is the seamless integration of appropriate internal and external data sources, which helps to identify and measure relevant performance metrics. In a BI architecture, as shown in Fig. 8.2, several different data sources can be used, including internal operational databases or external data sources. Typical operational databases in radiology are the picture archiving and communication system (PACS), electronic health

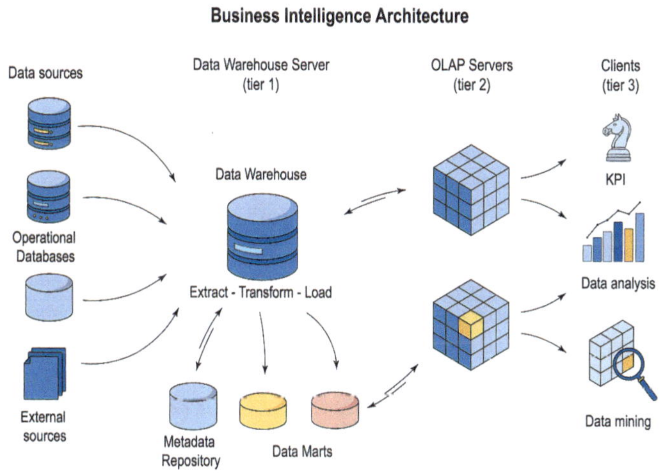

Business Intelligence Architecture

Fig. 8.2   Business intelligence (BI) architecture in radiology. BI in radiology consists of a number of distinct steps that are focused on extracting data from relevant data sources and subsequent storing in a data warehouse. From the data warehouse, several derivative databases (metadata repository and data marts) can be created for the purpose of performing analysis on subsets of the data. In modern BI architectures, data are stored in high-dimensional data cubes for online analytical processing (OLAP), making it possible to perform fast and real-time analysis of the data for the purpose of determining key performance indicators (KPIs) and dashboarding

records (EHR), physician scheduling systems, and more [10]. Depending on the specific performance metric, data needs to be gathered from one or more of these databases. This can, for instance, include, patient wait times, report turnaround time, diagnostic accuracy rates, equipment utilisation, resource utilisation, examination throughput, image acquisition time, stakeholder satisfaction surveys (patients, referring physicians, staff), and financial metrics (cost per examination, revenue generation, and budget adherence) [11]. It is unusual that a single system can provide the required data that can be used to determine all performance metrics. Therefore, it is more likely that several data sources need to be integrated and can write data to a single unified database, also referred to as a data warehouse. The process of extracting data from different operational databases, performing consistency checks, and storing into a data warehouse is also known as extraction, transforming and loading (ETL) [12]. With data stored in a data warehouse, it is possible to perform the required analysis on the data and calculate the performance metrics [13].

Although data can be queried directly from a data warehouse, it is also possible to have several derivative databases that contain a subset of the data warehouse, also known as data marts, from which data can be queried for analysis. Data warehouses often use relational database management systems, where data is stored in tables with a set of relationships applied to the data [12]. Although the use of relational databases is adequate for storing radiological and healthcare data, they are less suitable for performing ad hoc analysis because the results often require further processing, such as data cleaning, transformation, or aggregation, before they can be easily interpreted. Furthermore, scaling to larger databases can result in significantly longer analysis times. Another way of organising data which permits fast analysis and reporting is by using an online analytical process (OLAP). Using OLAP, data is aggregated into multidimensional data cubes instead of tables. [14] By connecting relational databases to OLAP, it is possible to perform ad-hoc queries and real-time analysis, permitting users to perform faster searches and analysis and generate on-demand graphical visualisations of data and reports.

8.3.2 Data for Evaluating AI Technology

While, like any other technological innovation, the impact of AI technology can be monitored using the proposed BI architecture, the diversity in technological implementations of currently available AI applications can complicate a streamlined approach to evaluate and monitor their performance. This is due to the inherent narrowness of current radiological AI applications, where a fully AI-enhanced radiological workflow will likely consist of multiple AI applications working in an orchestrated fashion. With the absence of standard integrations, AI applications can store relevant data that could be used for deriving performance metrics in different, sometimes even proprietary, databases. Furthermore, the way the medical institution decides to host AI technology will largely determine where relevant data on AI usage and performance will be stored. In this regard, evaluation and monitoring of AI can be performed on the level of the application itself and by using data from general operational databases (such as the PACS or EHR). When assessing the impact of AI on a particular workflow or radiological operation, for example, workflow efficiency, data from such general systems can be used to obtain relevant performance metrics. However, if the performance of specific AI applications requires to be monitored, then data from these general radiological or hospital systems might not yield the necessary information. This is particularly the case when AI applications are not directly integrated in clinical front-end systems such as the PACS or EHR. Instead, the database of the AI application itself is another data source that needs to be integrated in the BI framework. It is not uncommon for commercially available AI applications to have their own proprietary databases and software interfaces. These databases contain much relevant information on user interaction and usage of the application that can be relevant for specific performance metrics, though need to be separately integrated into the BI framework. Figure 8.3 illustrates an example integration of an AI application into the radiological workflow, featuring a continuous monitoring loop that tracks performance. This integration utilises connections with PACS and a duplicate database of the EHR system.

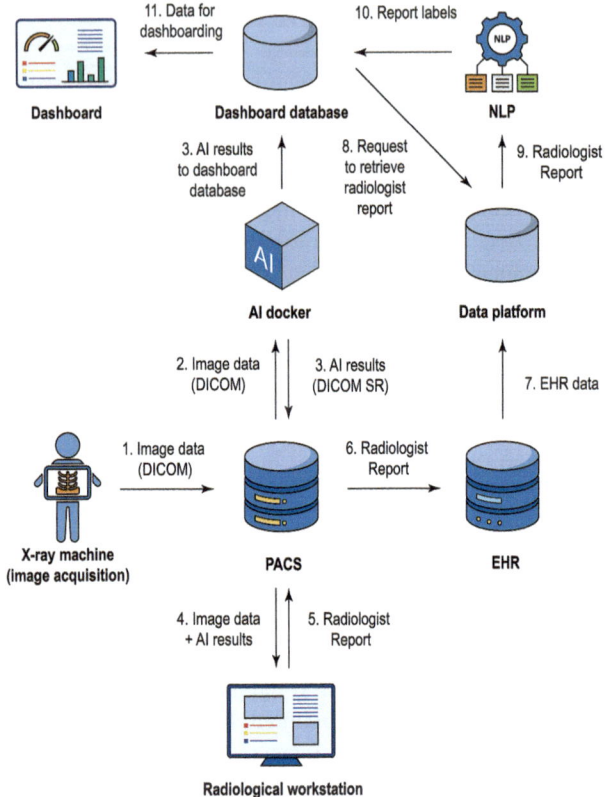

Fig. 8.3 Automated monitoring of an AI application in clinical routine. (1) After image acquisition, image data will be sent to the picture archiving and communications system (PACS). (2) Using inbound scripting, the PACS system selects appropriate imaging exams to be forwarded to the AI application. (3) The AI applications will process the image data and sends AI results back to the PACS and a dashboard database. (4) When the radiologist is ready to evaluate the images and create a report, relevant image data and AI results will be displayed on the radiological workstation. (5) After completion, the radiological report will be stored in the PACS system. (6) Subsequently, the report will be send to the electronic health records (EHR) system. (7) The data of the EHR system is copied to the data platform. (8) A retrieval request will be send to the data platform. (9) The radiological reports will be retrieved and processed using a natural language processing (NLP) algorithm. (10) Text labels will be stored together with the radiological report in the dashboard database. (11) The dashboard uses data from the dashboard database to display relevant metrics indicating the performance of the AI algorithm

Although such databases can be included as a potential data source in the BI framework, scaling the number of applications, where there is a need to integrate multiple standalone databases, will inevitably increase complexity. This issue of increased complexity is recognised by several providers of vendor neutral AI (VNAI) platforms. As mentioned previously, the VNAI platforms take on the role of hosting and orchestrating the use of multiple AI applications in clinical practice. This is particularly important if medical institutions choose to scale the number of applications for optimising their clinical practice. Given that these VNAI platforms in many cases store information on the use and sometimes even the performance of AI applications, these platforms themselves can act as a data source for a BI system. There are currently multiple platform providers that are able to store, analyse, and even display relevant performance metrics that can be used in a BI framework. Therefore, integrating data of such VNAI platforms with that of several clinical front-end systems, such as the EHR and PACS, is expected to provide a holistic overview of AI impact on the clinical workflow.

8.4   Analyse and Present

8.4.1 Key Performance Indicators

With clear and actionable objectives in place and having connected relevant data sources to the BI framework, it is of importance to define specific performance metrics that can be used to track specific radiological operations and processes. A specific type of performance indicators, the key performance indicators (KPIs), has been proven instrumental in monitoring critical operations across different fields, including in radiology. The distinguishing feature of KPIs is, when compared to other more general performance metrics, that they are always focused and quantifiable measures. Therefore, KPIs provide a means of quantitative assessment of performance of specific radiology operations, helping to steer development and monitor progress toward strategic goals and objectives [11]. Before setting up KPIs, it is important to determine what processes are relevant to monitor. The choice of KPI is therefore closely linked to the actual objective that is being considered. Generally, KPIs in radiology can be categorised into several overarching groups, namely quality and safety, stakeholder satisfaction, operations, and finance, from which several subcategories can be defined [15].

While AI applications can have an impact on several aspects of the radiological workflow, it can be helpful to prioritise KPIs of a specific category on which the AI application should have its intended effect on. For instance, if the bottleneck in a particular radiological workflow is efficiency, then KPIs focusing on radiology operations might be prioritised over finance, stakeholders, and quality. Furthermore, it is important not to define an excessive number of KPIs and attempt to measure too many aspects simultaneously. In other words, adhering to the sentiment expressed by the sociologist William Bruce Cameron, "Not everything that counts can be counted, and not everything that can be counted counts" serves as a valuable guiding principle in the establishment of KPIs. Indeed, having too many KPIs can impose a significant burden on involved staff and may be impractical or even impossible from a logistical standpoint [16]. Using a recent literature review by Moreira and Crispim, useful KPIs categorised according to the radiology value chain are provided in Table 8.1 [15]. In this table, Moreira and Crispim collected several KPIs in the radiology value chain found in other relevant literature [17–21].

After defining relevant KPIs for measuring specific aspects of radiology operations, it is important to assign responsibilities and determine the frequency at which they will be measured. Establishing clear roles and responsibilities is instrumental to create disciplined teams capable of systematically collecting KPI data. By forming several smaller teams, consisting of members from different disciplines and areas of expertise, dedicated to collecting data for specific KPIs serves the dual purpose of dividing the associated workload and creating a culture of awareness regarding the significance of these indicators to improve overall operations of the radiology department.

Table 8.1 Several key performance indicators (KPIs) in the radiology value chain that can be supported by the use of artificial intelligence (AI) applications. (Modified from Moreira and Crispim [15]). In this case, the KPIs are categorised into seven categories; (1) Accessibility to radiology services, (2) exam prescription adequacy, (3) exam process, (4) report, (5) results (6), safety (7), institutional citizenship (the way the Radiology Department participates or adds to the institution it belongs to). For each KPI category, examples on how AI can contribute to improving radiology services for that specific point are provided in the most right column

Category	Key performance indicator (KPI)	Use of artificial intelligence (AI) technology
Accessibility radiology services	1. Available slots for exam scheduling 2. Optimal timing between baseline and follow-up imaging 3. Mean time between ordering exam and having it scheduled 4. Percentage of tests scheduled and performed at a time and place that is convenient for the patient 5. Percentage of examinations and other complementary (non-radiological) examinations scheduled for the same day	• AI-driven resource forecasting and scheduling optimisation to increase equipment utilisation (predicting peak times and adjusting schedules accordingly) • Chatbots and AI-based communication platforms can streamline the process from ordering to scheduling exams, enhancing patient convenience • AI-based logistics optimisation can increase the percentage of tests and examinations scheduled for the same day, enhancing patient convenience

(continued)

Table 8.1 (continued)

Category	Key performance indicator (KPI)	Use of artificial intelligence (AI) technology
Exam prescription adequacy	1. Percentage of exams prescribed according to the reference guidelines/protocols 2. Percentage of duplicate, unnecessary or redundant prescribed exams 3. Radiologist participation rate in multidisciplinary meetings (discussion of cases of patients with other medical specialties) 4. Percentage of exam prescription with adequate clinical information	• AI-guided decision support systems can ensure exams are prescribed according to reference guidelines/protocols, reducing the number of unnecessary exams • AI models can identify patterns of duplicate or redundant exam prescriptions, taking clinical information into account • Facilitate the participation of radiologists in multidisciplinary meetings by organising and preparing relevant patient data efficiently using AI • AI-driven analysis of exam prescriptions for adequacy of clinical information day before the exam (highlighting relevant changes in patient condition) • Leveraging AI for dynamic guideline updates, ensuring prescriptions are always based on the latest clinical evidence

| Exam process | 1. Mean waiting time between arrival of the patient and start of the exam
2. Duration of radiological exam
3. Time elapsed between completion of exam and delivery of radiological report
4. Time between completion of exam and patient and leaving the radiology department
5. Number of required exam retakes
6. Average downtime between patient exams
7. Mean equipment downtime due to maintenance or technical issues
8. Percentage of patients receiving adequate information about the exam or procedure to be performed
9. Percentage of patients receiving a reminder (text message, phone call, etc.)
10. Percentage of patients attending the exam
11. For inpatients, mean time elapsed between leaving a ward and undergoing exam
12. Percentage of examinations performed according to established protocol | • Queue management systems powered by AI can reduce waiting times by optimising exam schedules
• AI can streamline exam duration through automated selection of imaging protocols and adjusting patient positioning
• Enhancement of image quality, reduction of scan time and/or radiation dose delivered to the patient using AI-based image reconstruction
• Using AI for the creation of synthetic image sets, omitting the need to have patients to undergo multiple radiological examinations on different imaging modalities
• Automated reporting tools to shorten the time between taking the exam and completing the report and reduce risk of oversight (enhance diagnostic accuracy)
• Predictive maintenance tools can decrease the downtime of equipment, improving operational efficiency
• Automated quality check after image acquisition (reducing retakes by providing feedback to technologists) |

(continued)

Table 8.1 (continued)

Category	Key performance indicator (KPI)	Use of artificial intelligence (AI) technology
Report	1. Percentage of peer-reviewed reports 2. Percentage of reports that meet established standards 3. Percentage of false positive or false negative findings 4. Percentage of reports that have the recommendations in the appropriate field 5. The error feedback rate to technologist and/or radiologists 6. Percentage of examinations in which the report was not made 7. Percentage of days with a 24-h radiologist coverage 8. Mean time to report and communicate critical findings 9. Percentage of patients who consulted their report 10. Percentage of patients to whom the report was explained and understood	• AI-assisted reporting to enhance the quality of reports and ensure they meet established standards • Use AI to detect (acute) finding to increase diagnostic accuracy and reduce report turnaround times • Automated quality control of report in the background in case of missed findings • AI can automate the placement of recommendations in reports and provide error feedback to technologists and radiologists • Use AI large language models (LLM) to rephrase medical jargon in report to ensure the report is understandable to the patient

Result	1. Percentage of referring physicians using radiological examination information for clinical management of patients	• AI-powered analytics can provide insights that make examination information more useful to prescribing physicians
	2. Percentage of exams that prevented the need of more expensive or invasive procedures	• Predictive models can assess the potential impact of exams on diagnosis or treatment, highlighting those that could prevent more invasive procedures
	3. Percentage exams that reduced inpatient length of stay	• Data analysis tools can identify correlations between exam outcomes and inpatient length of stay, supporting efforts to reduce it
	4. Percentage of satisfied patients	• AI-driven patient satisfaction analysis can provide feedback for service improvement
	5. Percentage of referring physicians satisfied with radiological services	• Use of AI for aggregating and visualising patient outcomes for better radiologist feedback, which can contribute to continuous learning and improvement
	6. Percentage of satisfied radiologists with delivered radiological services	

(continued)

Table 8.1 (continued)

Category	Key performance indicator (KPI)	Use of artificial intelligence (AI) technology
Safety	1. Percentage of exams with complication or incidents occurring during the exam 2. Percentage of critical exams delivered on time 3. Percentage of examinations with radiation dose registration and monitoring 4. The diagnostic protocols usage rate that involves the choice of exams that do not use radiation 5. Percentage of exams performed with recommended or lower radiation doses 6. The training rate about radiation protection 7. Percentage of examinations with appropriate safety checks were carried out prior to the patient's arrival	• AI algorithms can monitor and detect adverse events during exams, improving patient safety • Automated systems can ensure critical results are reported swiftly and efficiently • AI can support radiation dose monitoring and encourage the use of exams that minimise radiation exposure • Training modules powered by AI can enhance education on radiation protection and safety protocols
Institutional citizenship	1. The administrative meetings rate per year 2. The leadership positions rate on institution/hospital committees 3. Average time spent on administrative issues of the institution/hospital (minutes/week) 4. The marketing events rate to promote the health system 5. The certifications rate achieved by the department	• Data analytics can evaluate the impact of marketing events and guide strategies to promote the health system • AI-driven platforms can streamline the process for achieving certifications, ensuring continuous improvement • Potential of AI in identifying and predicting trends in radiology service demand, aiding strategic planning and resource allocation

8.4.2 Dashboards

After defining appropriate KPIs and connecting relevant data sources, it is important to present this information in an intuitive manner to facilitate informed decision-making. A common way to summarise information is by the use of dashboards. Dashboards play a pivotal role in visualising and understanding the impact of organisational and technological innovations, including that of AI, on radiological operations. They provide a direct and intuitive interface to different stakeholders by streamlining the presentation of complex data, making it possible to make informed decisions [22]. However, summarising a complex organisation like a radiology department using a dashboard is challenging. In pursuit of an optimal radiology dashboard, Kamari identified, by using a Delphi technique involving 30 radiologists, a total of 92 KPIs that were categorised in seven main areas for assessing radiology department performance. In subsequent steps, development of a robust dashboard design model encompassing crucial features like goal determination, alignment with organisational objectives, and security was discussed. A robust radiology dashboard demonstrating the performance of a department should encompass several essential features to provide comprehensive insights. Firstly, it should present KPIs clearly, offering a real-time overview of critical metrics related to safety, service, customer satisfaction, teaching and research, resource utilisation, financial performance, and workplace excellence. The dashboard must be user-customisable, allowing different stakeholders to tailor their views based on their specific needs. Integration with organisational goals and alignment with the department's objectives ensure that the presented data is strategically relevant. Flexibility in terms of data extraction, representation, and drill-down capabilities is crucial for a dynamic and responsive user experience. Additionally, the inclusion of security measures, effective visualisation techniques, and alert mechanisms enhance the overall utility of the dashboard. It thereby becomes a comprehensive tool for monitoring and optimising the performance of a radiology department, providing important information on the quality and effectiveness of radiological services delivered and its impact on patient care.

In addition to measuring the impact of AI on radiological operations, special focus should be given to systems that check the quality of the AI model itself over time. This also includes the detection of possible performance drifts that might arise. Data drift refers to the phenomenon where the model's input data changes over time, diverging from the data the model was originally trained on [23]. This divergence can be due to various factors such as changing patient populations, use of different imaging equipment, or changing image acquisition and reconstruction protocols. The importance of monitoring data drift lies in its potential to significantly degrade quality of the obtained AI results. In practical situations, understanding and addressing data drift are crucial to ensure that AI models continue to perform optimally and remain relevant. Integrating data drift detection into quality control dashboards is essential for maintaining well-functioning AI-enhanced radiological workflows. Therefore, dashboards should ideally include KPIs that also focus on measuring data drift, such as changes in data distribution over time or discrepancies between predicted and actual outcomes. By presenting these metrics in an accessible and intuitive manner, it becomes possible to identify performance issues promptly, ensuring that AI-driven processes remain accurate, effective, and safe. This proactive approach to quality control facilitates informed decision-making and supports the sustainable integration of AI technologies in a post-implementation setting.

8.5   Evaluate and Decide

Following the collection, analysis, and presentation of data, the subsequent task is to determine whether adjustments to particular radiology operations are warranted. At this stage, department management will need to leverage the information provided by the KPIs to make informed decisions aimed at further optimising the radiological workflow. This requires the simultaneous interpretation of information that different KPIs provide and use them for guidance to make strategic changes to enhance efficiency, quality, diagnostic accuracy, and patient care. The effectiveness of this phase lies in its ability to transform data-driven insights into tangible actions, thereby closing the loop of the BI cycle and setting the stage for continuous improvement. By integrating a comprehensive evaluation of KPIs with a strategic decision making process, radiology departments can adeptly navigate the complexities of their operations, ensuring that each decision is aligned with overarching organisational goals and contributes to the refinement of the radiological workflow.

8.5.1 Performance Management System

Before strategic decisions can be made using the collected KPI data, it is of importance how to source information from this data. Therefore, creating an overview of KPIs measured and the intricate interconnections is a first important step that should be undertaken. Having such an overview is vital for monitoring the performance of a complex organisation that requires the use of numerous KPIs. A performance management system enables the aggregation and analysis of KPIs, facilitating informed decision-making regarding various radiological processes. Many organisations and enterprises use performance management systems to monitor specific operations. Among the various performance management systems available, the Balanced Scorecard (BSC) approach stands out as a widely recognised method. It is particularly effective in identifying and illustrating the relationships between different performance metrics. This enables organisations to track, evaluate, and enhance their overall performance in a comprehensive manner. Originally, the BSC model, as described by Kaplan and Norton, works by taking four key perspectives into account, namely financial performance, customers, internal processes and operations, and learning and growth [24]. Relevant performance metrics are categorised in these overarching principles that are considered to be important for organisational success.

Over the years, subsequent iterations of the first-generation BSC model yielded second- and third-generation models where KPIs are more explicitly linked to strategic goals and objectives of the organisation instead of the aforementioned four key perspectives. Another noteworthy feature within the third-generation BSC models is the introduction of KPI trees, which is a specific type of third-generation strategy map. A KPI tree provides a structured overview of the logical relationships between different KPIs and their connections to overarching strategic objectives [16]. The advantage of this type of visualisation is that it provides an intuitive understanding on how KPIs contribute to broader goals and objectives of the organisation. A KPI tree typically consists of different layers, constituting high level goals and objectives, strategic outcomes or focus aligned with each strategic objective, and KPIs connected to each of the strategic outcomes [16]. This can be particularly useful for monitoring the impact of AI applications in radiology, where the implementation of many different solutions in different aspects of the clinical workflow becomes complex and difficult to track. Figure 8.4 depicts a radiology KPI tree showing an example of a strategic objective focusing on the efficiency and diagnostic quality of chest X-rays.

Within each layer of the KPI tree are different elements that support the next layer of abstraction. Lines between different elements illustrate connections and the logical relationships and dependencies between different KPIs and outcomes. With many different modifications to the workflow, for example, due to the integration of different AI applications, illustrating these connections offers managers and stakeholders insight on how various technologies influence different aspects of the workflow. Although KPI trees are principally easily readable and explainable, creating them can be non-intuitive and demanding, particularly when comparing to earlier generations of BSC models.

8.5.2 Rethinking Radiological Workflows—The Theory of Constraints

Having established a robust performance management system and gathered relevant KPI data, the responsibility falls on decision-makers to determine the necessary actions. This involves interpreting the KPI data to draw suitable conclusions. When AI-driven

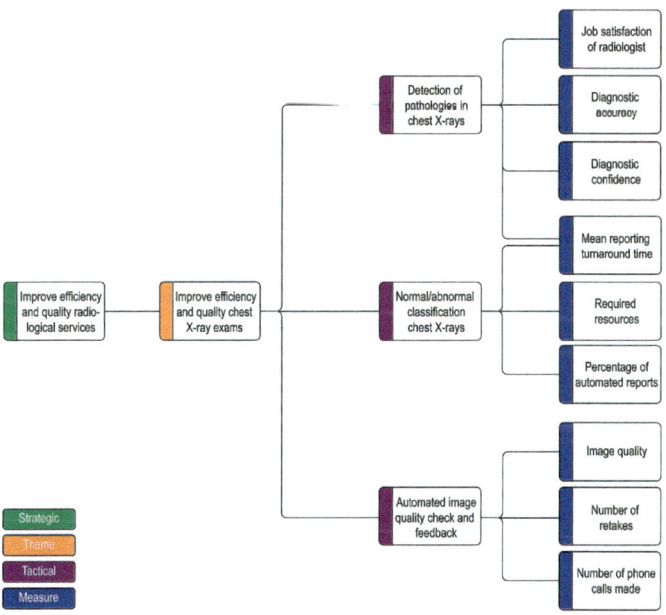

Fig. 8.4 Key performance indicator (KPI) tree showing the relation between a strategic objective and change initiatives together with KPIs. From left to right are three different layers of abstraction (strategic, theme, tactical, and measure). On the far left is the strategic objective (focusing on improving efficiency and quality of radiological services). The strategic objective is supported by different themes. Within each theme, different change initiatives are proposed that are supported by their associated KPIs. In this example, a theme that focuses on the improved efficiency and quality of chest X-ray exams is shown. The theme is supported by tactical change initiatives focusing on AI implementation (an automated AI-based quality check system, automated normal/abnormal detection, and AI-based detection of findings on chest X-rays). The impact of tactical change initiatives is measured by several relevant KPIs

initiatives do not meet their expected performance levels, a thorough evaluation is essential to identify the root causes, which may include issues with data quality, algorithm efficiency, user adoption, or clinical alignment. Such an evaluation should prompt a strategic discussion on prioritising adjustments within the AI implementation roadmap. Departments may look into organising user training programmes to boost adoption rates, or modify the AI application to enhance performance or better align with clinical requirements. Collaboration with AI vendors for technical support, algorithm retraining with tailored datasets, and receiving updates are also vital components. While focusing on the performance of an individual application is beneficial, it can be worthwhile to consider the entire workflow of a specific radiological service to get a broader perspective. It is important to recognise that if the performance of a single application does not deliver the expected benefits, employing a combination of multiple AI applications might. For instance, the positive impact of AI applications that improve reporting efficiency could be constrained by the department's production capacity. By introducing additional AI applications aimed at reducing image acquisition times or otherwise increasing the capacity for scaling the volume of radiological examinations, alongside the initial application, the department might achieve the desired increase in production rates.

By viewing the entire workflow holistically and treating radiological processes as interconnected rather than as isolated steps, decision-makers can employ the principles of the "Theory of Constraints"—a renowned methodology in supply chain logistics—to improve radiological workflow efficiency [25]. The Theory of Constraints posits that every system has at least one bottleneck that limits its overall performance, and improving the system involves identifying and addressing this bottleneck. In the context of radiology, applying the five steps of this theory—(1) identifying the system's constraint, (2) exploiting the constraint to its fullest, (3) subordinating everything else to the decision made in step two, (4) elevating the system's constraint, and (5) returning to the first step if the constraint has shifted—can lead to significant enhancements in workflow efficiency. By systematically applying these steps, radiology departments can ensure that resources are optimally allocated, workflows are streamlined, and patient throughput is maximised, all while maintaining or improving diagnostic accuracy [26]. This strategic approach enables departments to continuously adapt and improve, leveraging AI innovations to overcome operational challenges and meet evolving clinical demands.

8.6   Action

8.6.1   Project Management

Creating and executing an action plan to improve radiological operations is a critical phase that follows the evaluation and decision-making process. The success of this phase depends on several key considerations, each playing a pivotal role in ensuring the plan's alignment with the department's goals and the broader organisational context. Firstly, the importance of clear and effective communication cannot be overstated. It is essential to articulate the action plan's objectives, expected outcomes, and the roles of different team members transparently and concisely. This ensures that all stakeholders are on the same page and take ownership and commitment to the project's success. Establishing a multidisciplinary team that includes radiologists, technicians, administrative staff, and IT professionals facilitates a comprehensive approach to implementing the plan, ensuring that all operational, clinical, and technological aspects are considered.

Moreover, choosing the right project management methodology is crucial to the plan's successful execution [9]. While traditional project management approaches offer structured and linear steps, agile methodologies may be more suitable for projects requiring flexibility and iterative progress, especially when implementing AI innovations or technological upgrades. Agile methods allow for rapid adjustments based on feedback and changing needs, promoting continuous improvement and collaboration among team members. However, the chosen methodology should resonate with the department's culture and operational dynamics [27]. Implementing project management tools and software can enhance coordination and track progress and maintain accountability throughout the project's lifecycle. Additionally, setting up regular check-ins and review meetings helps in monitoring progress against milestones, addressing challenges promptly, and adjusting strategies as needed. It is crucial that the action plan is not only ambitious but also realistic, with achievable milestones set against a clearly defined timeline.

8.6.2 Structured Problem Solving

In addition to using a fitting project management system, the incorporation of structured problem-solving methodologies can assist in offering flexibility when moving to the project's execution phase. Particularly in complex technological and organisational environments where systems depend on many different pieces acting together, things tend to go differently than expected. Structured problem-solving methodologies provide a systematic approach to identifying, analysing, and resolving issues that may impede the successful execution of an action plan. One widely recognised framework is the Plan-Do-Check-Act (PDCA) cycle, also known as the Shewhart cycle, which encourages continuous improvement by planning actions, implementing them, checking the outcomes, and acting on what has been learned [28]. Similarly, the Six Sigma methodology focuses on reducing variability and defects through a data-driven approach, utilising the Define, Measure, Analyse, Improve, and Control (DMAIC) process [29]. These methodologies not only facilitate a deep understanding of operational challenges but also create an environment where solutions are based on empirical evidence and rigorous analysis.

Implementing such structured problem-solving techniques ensures that decisions are not made in isolation but are backed by a thorough investigation and understanding of the underlying issues. This disciplined approach is crucial for tackling complex challenges inherent in radiological operations. Moreover, it empowers teams to break down seemingly insurmountable problems into manageable components, enabling targeted interventions that are more likely to yield positive results. By integrating structured problem-solving methodologies and a suitable project management system into the execution phase of the action plan, radiology departments can significantly enhance their strategic thinking, innovation, and resilience to operational challenges, laying a robust foundation for the adoption of new technologies and continuous improvement in radiological services and patient care.

8.7   Conclusions

This chapter underscores the critical role of BI in enhancing radiological operations through the strategic implementation of AI. As radiology departments continue to integrate advanced AI technologies, the importance of a robust BI framework cannot be overstated. BI systems enable the effective monitoring and evaluation of AI's impact, helping to optimise workflows, improve patient care, and meet organisational objectives. By establishing clear success criteria aligned with the broader goals of the healthcare institution, radiology departments can leverage BI to identify inefficiencies, guide resource allocation, and enhance operational decisions.

Furthermore, the integration of AI demands continuous adaptation and alignment with evolving healthcare landscapes. The use of performance metrics and KPIs within a well-structured BI framework allows for the precise assessment of AI's contributions to radiological practices. Ultimately, by embracing BI principles, radiology departments can not only fulfil immediate operational goals but also pave the way for sustainable innovation and enhanced patient outcomes in an increasingly data-driven era. This chapter sets the stage for radiology departments to harness the full potential of AI and BI, driving forward the transformation of radiological services in the modern healthcare environment.

References

1. Rezazade Mehrizi MH, van Ooijen P, Homan M. Applications of artificial intelligence (AI) in diagnostic radiology: a technography study. Eur Radiol. 2021;31:1805–11.
2. Kelly BS, et al. Radiology artificial intelligence: a systematic review and evaluation of methods (RAISE). Eur Radiol. 2022;32:7998–8007.
3. Dedić N, Stanier C. Measuring the success of changes to existing business intelligence solutions to improve business intelligence reporting. In: Lecture notes in business information processing. Cham: Springer International Publishing; 2016. p. 225–36.
4. Froze R. Business intelligence for beginners!: An easy to follow guide to data integration, analytics & more. Createspace Independent Publishing Platform; 2016.
5. Sherman R. Business intelligence guidebook: from data integration to analytics. Newnes; 2014.
6. Kim B, Romeijn S, van Buchem M, Mehrizi MHR, Grootjans W. A holistic approach to implementing artificial intelligence in radiology. Insights Imaging. 2024;15:22.
7. Huebner C, Flessa S. Strategic management in healthcare: a call for long-term and systems-thinking in an uncertain system. Int J Environ Res Public Health. 2022;19:8617.
8. Birchall D. Benchmarking in radiology: apples and oranges? Br J Radiol. 2010;83:1–3.
9. Larson DB, Mickelsen LJ. Project management for quality improvement in radiology. Am J Roentgenol. 2015;205:W470–7.
10. Shah A, Muddana PS, Halabi S. A review of core concepts of imaging informatics. Cureus. 2022;14:e32828.
11. Abujudeh HH, Kaewlai R, Asfaw BA, Thrall JH. Quality initiatives: key performance indicators for measuring and improving radiology department performance. Radiographics. 2010;30:571–80.
12. Prevedello LM, Andriole KP, Hanson R, Kelly P, Khorasani R. Business intelligence tools for radiology: creating a prototype model using open-source tools. J Digit Imaging. 2010;23:133–41.
13. Liman L, May B, Fette G, Krebs J, Puppe F. Using a clinical data warehouse to calculate and present key metrics for the radiology department: implementation and performance evaluation. JMIR Med Inform. 2023;11:e41808.
14. Haque W, Urquhart B, Berg E, Dhanoa R. Using business intelligence to analyze and share health system infrastructure data in a rural health authority. JMIR Med Inform. 2014;2:e16.
15. Moreira A, Crispim J. Key performance indicators for value-based reimbursement in radiology: a review. Procedia Comput Sci. 2023;219:1208–15.

16. Smith B. KPI checklists: develop meaningful, trusted, KPIs and reports using step-by-step checklists. Metric Press; 2013.
17. Boland GW, et al. Report of the ACR's economics committee on value-based payment models. J Am Coll Radiol. 2017;14:6–14.
18. Patel S. Value management program: performance, quantification, and presentation of imaging value-added actions. J Am Coll Radiol. 2015;12:239–48.
19. Sarwar A, Boland G, Monks A, Kruskal JB. Metrics for radiologists in the era of value-based health care delivery. Radiographics. 2015;35:866–76.
20. European Society of Radiology (ESR). ESR concept paper on value-based radiology, vol. 8. Insights Imaging; 2017. p. 447–54.
21. Heller RE 3rd, et al. Quality measures and pediatric radiology: suggestions for the transition to value-based payment. Pediatr Radiol. 2017;47:776–82.
22. Karami M. A design protocol to develop radiology dashboards. Acta Inform Med. 2014;22:341–6.
23. Sahiner B, Chen W, Samala RK, Petrick N. Data drift in medical machine learning: implications and potential remedies. Br J Radiol. 2023;96:20220878.
24. Kaplan RS, Norton DP. The balanced scorecard—measures that drive performance. Harv Bus Rev. 1992;70:71–9.
25. Goldratt EM. Critical chain. North River Press; 1997.
26. MacDonald SLS, et al. Measuring and managing radiologist workload: application of lean and constraint theories and production planning principles to planning radiology services in a major tertiary hospital. J Med Imaging Radiat Oncol. 2013;57:544–50.
27. Rawson JV, Davis MA. Change management: a framework for adaptation of the change management model. IISE Trans Healthc Syst Eng. 2023;13:198–204. https://doi.org/10.1080/24725579.2023.2201959.
28. Deming WE. Out of the crisis, reissue. MIT Press; 2018.
29. George M, Maxey J, Rowlands D, Upton M. The lean six sigma pocket toolbook: a quick reference guide to 70 tools for improving quality and speed: a quick reference guide to 70 tools for improving quality and speed: a quick reference guide to 70 tools for improving quality and speed. McGraw Hill Professional; 2004.

The Impact of AI on Radiology Reporting

9

J. M. Nobel 🔘

Key Points
- It is important to first understand the radiological reporting process, including the principles of standardization and structured reporting, before implementing NLP tools like LLMs in the reporting workflow.
- The use of LLMs in the radiological reporting process can improve the radiological report.
- When implementing AI into the reporting process, it is important to stay focused on the main goal: producing a readable and accurate radiological report.
- In the near future, it will be important to address issues concerning direct information transfer between algorithms for image analysis and NLP-based algorithms.

J. M. Nobel (✉)
Department of Radiology and Nuclear Medicine,
Maastricht University Medical Center+, Maastricht, The Netherlands

GROW Research Institute for Oncology and Reproduction,
Maastricht University, Maastricht, The Netherlands
e-mail: martijn.nobel@mumc.nl

© The Author(s), under exclusive license to Springer Nature Switzerland AG 2024
E. Ranschaert et al. (eds.), *AI Implementation in Radiology*, Imaging Informatics for Healthcare Professionals,
https://doi.org/10.1007/978-3-031-68942-0_9

9.1   Radiology Reporting on a Cross Road

The radiological report is the main output of the radiologist and is considered the golden standard in radiology communication [1–5]. It thereby is a medicolegal document [6–8] and important aspects about a particular entity should be described by the reporter in this report [1–5, 9, 10]. Therefore, the radiological report is very important in radiological practice. In addition, it is also very important in the clinical process, as it is the translational step between the medical question and the interpretation of the findings on the radiological examination [11, 12].

In the last decades, digitalization in healthcare, the introduction of the Picture Archive and Communication System (PACS) and Radiology Information System (RIS) changed radiology practice dramatically [12–15]. This led to changes in the way of reporting and allowed for better access to the radiological report by the referring clinician and general practitioner [2, 12]. The integration of speech recognition in radiology practice has enhanced the reporting process even more, as direct and faster reporting into the PACS became possible [16–20]. However, the radiological report and the reporting process are still the same.

The introduction of Artificial Intelligence (AI) enhanced opportunities in radiology even further and can be seen as one of the largest game-changers of this century [21–27]. AI is already available for image interpretation, such as radiomics [28–30]. Also, multiple tools are being offered to detect all kinds of abnormalities, like, for instance, fracture detection, pulmonary nodule, or pneumonia detection or brain hemorrhage detection that should improve accuracy and efficiency of the reporter [31].

AI focusing on free text and language spoken by humans (natural language) is called Natural Language Processing (NLP). Recently, AI made significant steps in the field of language processing, leading to new possibilities and applications in the field of radiological reporting, ultimately resulting in an improved radiological report.

This chapter will focus on the reporting process in radiology in general, the most recent attempts to improve it and the potential impact of NLP in this field.

9.2   Improving Radiology Reporting

9.2.1   Reporting Process

Instead of diving into the possibilities of NLP, it is important to stay focused on our goal: improving radiology reporting. The reporting process is highly complex and only little has changed in the way of reporting since the beginning of reporting in radiology [1–4, 6, 10, 11, 32]. Mostly, the radiological report still consists of free text.

The radiological reporting process starts with a clinical question that will be answered by the radiologist in the report, after the examination indication is set and the examination has been performed by the technician. Two main items in this process are considered to lead to a good report: (1) accurate content and (2) readable structure (Fig. 9.1.).

In search for a better radiological report, an abundance of reporting guidelines are known [1–16, 32–37]. In addition, the ongoing call for standardization and the even more recent move toward structured reporting are perfect examples of the wish (or need) to change the reporting process. Recently, structured reporting in particular has been promoted by radiological societies, in an attempt to improve the accuracy and readability of the radiological report [17, 18, 38–40] (Fig. 9.2).

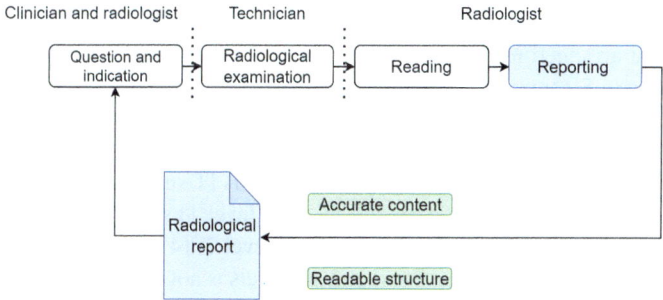

Fig. 9.1 Radiological reporting process

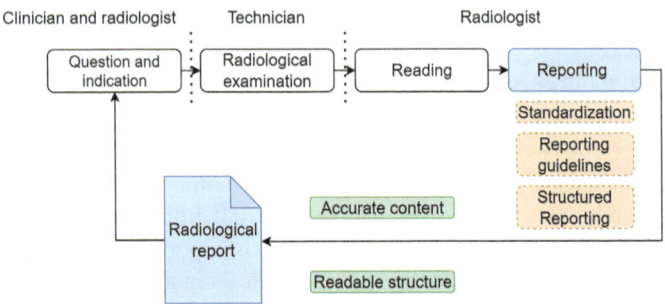

Fig. 9.2 Radiological reporting process and tools to increase the value of the radiological report; standardization, reporting guidelines, and structured reporting

9.2.1.1 Standardized Reporting and Structured Reporting

To understand the possibilities of NLP in the radiological reporting process properly, it is important to know the conceptual difference between standardized reporting and structured reporting. At this moment, various assumptions of what involves standardized reporting and structured reporting are circulating in literature and therefore a clear distinction between both concepts and understanding of standardized reporting and structured reporting is lacking.

It is postulated that standardized reporting is about streamlining the medical content of the radiological report [41]. As such, it is important to all use the same vocabulary and the same grading scales like, for instance, the RADS family [42]. Separately, structured reporting deals with how this medical content is imported and arranged into the radiological report [41, 43, 44]. A distinction in SR type can be made based on its level of IT-infrastructure that is demanded to implement. As an example, a simple template should not necessarily be supported by any IT tool, whereas a drop down menu or specific pick-list needs IT support. As such a template not supported by any IT tool (level 1) should be distinguished from a dedicated IT solution (level 2) [41, 43, 44].

The main difference between both levels is not the medical content of the radiological report itself or the lay-out of the report, which can look similar, but the way of storing the data, since only structured stored data is directly usable for data mining purposes whereas free text is not. This is because structured data will fully fit a data model, hereby meeting the FAIR principles (Findable, Accessible, Interoperable, and Reusable) [45]. Hence, structured data is retrievable (Findable), because it is placed in a particular location. Because the data on that location is defined and the information is known, it can facilitate data mining. This is in contrast to a free text template which consists of standard sentences or predefined text in a predefined order. This free text data does not have a particular location and not every location contains the same type of information, so it will not be suitable to be reused directly. This highlights the difference between free text data stored in a standardized structured manner (level 1) and structured stored data (level 2).

- **Standardization** is about streamlining the medical content of the radiological report.

- **Structured reporting** is about importing and arranging the medical content in the radiological report by means of IT [41].

9.3   Data Mining and Natural Language Processing in the Reporting Process

Currently, enormous quantities of patient data—patient follow ups, blood results as well as their medical history—are stored digitally in the medical Electronic Health Record (EHR) [43, 44, 46, 47]. This also includes the radiological report. This medical information can potentially be used for many tasks, like education and research but also in workflow improvement, quality assurance and even support the diagnostic process. However, most of this information is left unused, as it is stored as free text and in an unstructured manner and, as data retrieval of unstructured data is very laborious, it is not easy to (re)use [41, 43, 44, 46–48]. This is also true for data of the radiological report, which is mostly written as unstructured free text and therefore not easy to be reused directly in the reporting process or at a later stage for research purposes.

> Data Mining: The process of searching and analyzing data by means of computed power in order to find specific endpoints or correlations.

Data mining [28, 45, 46, 49] is considered to be a solution for processing and analyzing all kinds of data. By means of computed power, it is possible to search for specific data or correlations in the available data. Due to increased availability of computable power and the availability of AI, it is possible to search enormous amounts of data and as a result we can explore the capabilities of data mining in its largest form.

Text mining or NLP is a subtype of AI and can be used for searching, processing, and analyzing all kinds of text files, as, for instance, the radiological report [41, 48, 50–53]. As stated in Sect. 9.1 (Radiology reporting on a cross road), NLP is AI that is focusing on free text and language spoken by humans (natural language).

> Natural Language Processing: AI that is focusing on free text and language spoken by humans (natural language) is called Natural Language Processing (NLP).

When returning to the reporting process, NLP is the latest development that can improve the radiological process in search for a better radiological report. Where standardization is about streamlining the medical content and structured reporting deals with how and where information should be placed, NLP is seen as a game-changer capable of doing all kinds of things in the entire reporting process. NLP can potentially be of added value in producing or analyzing the final or preliminary report, it can help with making a particular diagnosis or can add a particular analysis of the content of the report and it can assist in retrieving additional information of the patient, already known from the electronic health record (EHR). For now the possibilities seem to have an enormous potential [52–55], but the same was true about structured reporting [1, 32, 33, 39, 44], where implementation still lags behind expectations. Therefore, it is important to

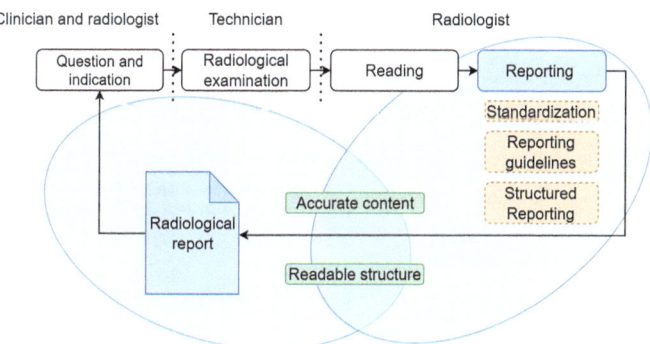

Fig. 9.3 Radiological reporting process with the added locations to implement NLP

understand capabilities of NLP as well as how and where in the reporting process it is best to implement. When looking at the radiological reporting process (Fig. 9.2), NLP can potentially be added on all different steps in the process. However, the main locations to improve the radiological report are (1) at the location of "reporting" or (2) at the end of the cycle at the "radiological report" and will be explained further in the next paragraph (Fig. 9.3).

9.4   Understanding Natural Language Processing

9.4.1   Natural Language Understanding (NLU) vs. Natural Language Generation (NLG)

If we go back in history for only 10 years, NLP was theoretically subdivided into Natural Language Generation (NLG) and Natural Language Understanding (NLU) (Fig. 9.4) [56, 57]. NLG was used to generate text, whereas NLU was used to understand text. For both it was necessary to have structured input, as in NLP the phrase "garbage in, is garbage out" is applicable. Hence, the more standardized and structured available data is, the better the NLP can process the input allowing for the most accurate outcome.

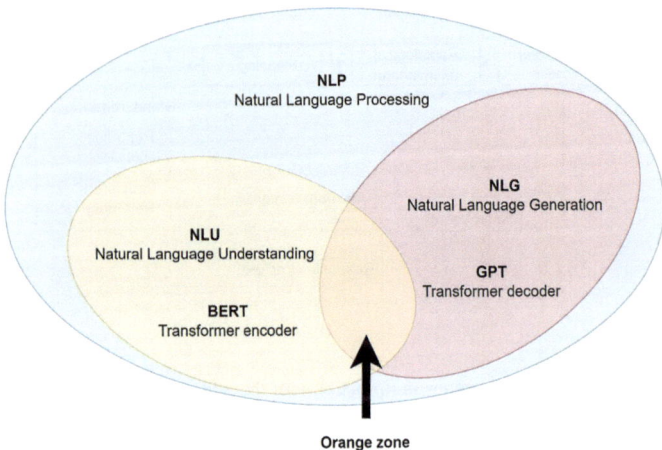

Orange zone

Fig. 9.4 The total field of Natural Language Processing (NLP), consisting of Natural Language Generation (NLG) and Natural Language Understanding (NLU). Later replaced by Bidirectional Encoder Representations from Transformer (BERT) and Generative Pretrained Transformer (GPT). Orange zone; LLMs with encoder and decoder capabilities

9.4.2   The Introduction of Transformers Like Bidirectional Encoder Representations from Transformers (BERT) and Generative Pretrained Transformer (GPT)

Only 5 years later, the field of text mining evolved, and due to the introduction of "transformers" terminology in NLP changed. As such NLG was replaced by transformer decoder and NLU was replaced by transformer encoder algorithms [58, 59]. As such, for understanding the transformer architecture, it is easiest to assume that the transformer decoder has roughly the same functionality as NLG and the encoder algorithms the same as NLU. The most well-known transformers are Bidirectional Encoder Representations from Transformers (BERT) and Generative Pretrained Transformer (GPT) [58, 59]. BERT can be seen as an encoder, GPT as a decoder. If we return to Fig. 9.4, we can add BERT to the yellow NLU balloon and GPT to the red NLG balloon.

In addition, transferred learning was introduced which made it possible to reuse knowledge learned by means of AI in other tasks or other fields than in the field of interest. For example, knowledge about size recognition, names, or negations trained on free available data could be used on medical information as well. Due to the introduction of transferred learning the necessity of having annotated data and supervised training in all separate settings became less important and the functionality of algorithms like BERT and GPT increased rapidly [58, 59]. In addition, many new versions or expanded Large Language Models (LLMs) are known, such as RoBERTa, DeBERTa, BERTje, and CamemBERT as encoders and, for instance, GPT-2, GPT-3, GPT-J, and ChatGPT as decoder transformers [58, 59].

Meanwhile, the algorithms became so hungry and the available data so enormous that due to the self-learning aspect of the transformers, the encoding and decoding (=understanding and generating) part of the spectrum of text mining became less important. For instance, ChatGPT is now capable of generating *and* understanding text– knowing that it is originally a decoding tool.

Large language model is an artificial intelligence system that is trained on billions of words derived from articles, books, and other internet-based content [58].

Nowadays, also several LLMs are becoming multimodal (M-LLMs), highlighting more extensive tasks [59–61]. When we return to Fig. 9.4, the orange zone points out the location where the yellow and red balloon overlap; this is the zone where LLMs are capable of understanding and generating text; the implementational possibilities seem to be endless.

9.4.3 Reporting Process

Returning to the reporting process, the main locations to improve the radiological report are (1) at the location of "reporting" (by helping the reporter) generating text or (2) at the end of the cycle

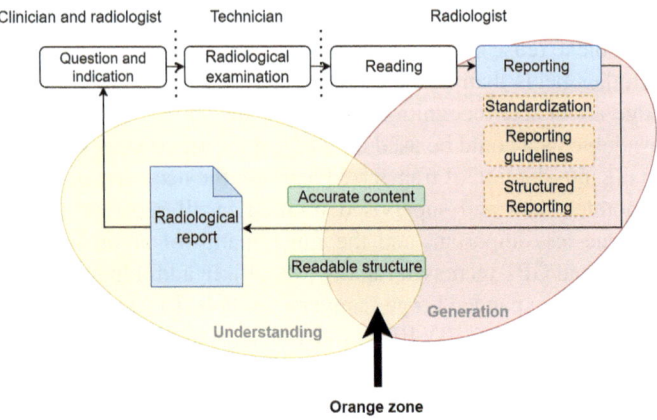

Fig. 9.5 Radiology reporting process and tools to increase the value of the radiological report; standardization, reporting guidelines, structured reporting, and natural language processing via data extraction and processing

at the "radiological report" by understanding (extracting, processing, and structuring) the text of the radiological report. One can imagine that free text reports will benefit most from text understanding, while text generation is best when data is standardized and structured (Fig. 9.5.). However, when we enter the orange zone of LLMs, such as ChatGPT, the distinction between tasks is becoming less clear because the algorithms are capable of doing multiple things at the same time. When such tools are implemented into the radiological reporting process, only the content accuracy and the readability of the final report remain important.

9.5   NLP in Radiology Research and Clinical Practice

9.5.1   Structured Reporting

As NLP in radiology reporting is able to process the free text radiological report, it can assist in improving the reporting process and thereby in making the radiological report itself.

In this context, NLP can be used to structure unstructured free text data so it can be processed and analyzed, and thereby function as a replacement for structured reporting. After all, instead of using structured reporting in which textual data is inserted and stored in a structured way, NLP can also accomplish this structured storage using computing power without the help of the reporter. By doing so, text mining can facilitate all kinds of post processing concerning report content by understanding text, generating text, or by doing both. However, we have to keep in mind that standardized and structured input will still give the highest outcome accuracy. Hence, despite the AI tools that exist, it is best to have FAIR data than to make data FAIR.

9.5.2   Standardized Reporting

As NLP is capable of structuring free text, it can also help in standardizing the content of the radiological report by suggesting the correct words or nomenclature used in a particular setting. For instance, helping the reporter to adjust to the correct terms in thoracic imaging as suggested by the Fleischner Society [62]. In addition, it can be used to assist radiological residents by finding the correct words or phrases used in a particular context.

9.5.3   Overall Research

Nowadays, NLP in healthcare is mainly applied in research settings, and many applications, especially implementation of ChatGPT, are being discussed [52–55]. One can imagine that applying and understanding LLMs in a research setting by selecting a particular patient category or when one or a few particular (standardized) entries need to be found, is already possible. However, when the demands are becoming more strict, or as the algorithm needs to include all patients or find all entries, the accuracy needs to be higher and is it more difficult to train. Nevertheless, there are many tasks that will benefit from this relatively "shallow" NLP usage in healthcare research already.

In radiology, several examples are known in which text under-standing applications are used to mine the radiological report, which mainly focus on query-based case retrieval or cohort build-ing, diagnostic support, clinical support, or surveillance or quality assessment [52–55]. There are already clinical practice tools available that are able to alert a referring clinician when an impor-tant outcome, such as an acute appendicitis, pneumonia, or throm-boembolic disease is being diagnosed [63–66]. In addition, it is possible to make a real-time recommendation for additional X-ray or MRI to be made, when a particular fracture is described in the radiological report [67]. This is also possible for antibiotics rec-ommendation when pneumonia is diagnosed [68, 69]. Such text understanding tools can also be used in the oncological setting by ascertaining oncological outcomes of regular follow-ups, tumor recurrence rates, for follow-up of acute oncological findings or for oncological classification or cancer registries [70–78].

Text generation tools can be seen as the little brother of text understanding tools, but with the increased possibilities of LLMs such as GPT and BERT models they have an enormous potential [52–55, 58, 59]. When focusing on text generation, research is being performed like NLP tools that are used for quality control, stating automated report impressions, construction of layperson reports, or checking the report content [52–55, 58, 59]. However, almost all of them are still implemented in research settings. No real implementation of LLMs that are capable of understanding and generating text is known at this moment; however, this prob-ably will change very fast.

9.6 Important Considerations Concerning Implementation of NLP

9.6.1 Current Situation

The aforementioned gives us the background information needed to understand the past, but also understand the future of reporting in radiology. As large language models are becoming more widely available in our digital world, the amount of LLMs sufficient to be used in healthcare is still limited [79]. This is not unusual, as medical data is not freely available and this type of data is relatively scarce. Whereas LLMs have a fairly high learning curve in daily life (public domain), this is not (yet) the case in healthcare. Though, the expectation is that, due to the current increased interest in NLP, applications and the possibility of transferred learning in the field of NLP, this for sure will enhance the speed of implementation.

However, an important constraint of implementing NLP tools in healthcare is that the acceptance of errors is low, as compared to other fields. As a consequence, implementation of NLP in case of decision-making or reporting results can only be done when the NLP tool has a high accuracy or, and less difficult, when the algorithm is supervised in daily practice. The lack of availability at this moment and the accuracy demands are two main limitations of NLP and its implementation in healthcare [52, 53, 55, 80].

9.6.2   User Interface as Reporting Tool

Perhaps a sidestep, but even as important as implementing AI or NLP, is the interaction between reporter and the tool. Currently, all kinds of AI implementation and tools exist, both on imaging and on textual data, and many different tools can run in clinical practice and on different (digital) locations. As a consequence, there should be a digital location where the reporter is aided by the AI and where the AI can be checked by the reporter. This location can be a so-called Graphical User Interface (GUI). This is ideally situated in or should at least be linked to the PACS, RIS, and ideally also to the EHR. In addition, speech recognition should also be integrated to allow for an environment in which the combination of reporter and AI can flourish. This environment should centralize the reporter and relieve their work with the assistance of AI.

However, one important notification should be made in this new reporter-AI relation. The environment should be vendor independent or perhaps vendor neutral in a way that every AI tool can be used by every reporter on every vendor software. Because of the rapid changes in the world of AI, and especially in the world of NLP, it is no longer possible to be strictly bound to one particular vendor and what they can offer. This GUI should also be the location on which analysis and tooling can be checked and analyzed in order to control the results and validate the AI tools over time as upgrades will have different outcomes.

Speech recognition should be integrated as well, because analysis of the textual data can be facilitated by implementation of NLP. In the future, it might be possible to analyze speech input before it is placed into the report. By doing so it is possible that the output is rephrased by the AI tool or that only facts (e.g., liver tumor and its size) should be mentioned while NLP constructs a sentence.

For now, it is possible to start adding information from a particular AI tool to the radiological report. However, the landing location of this information as well as the quality control of the content and its reusability in one particular system will be an ongoing process of reshaping functionality. Of course, the aforementioned is true for both imaging and textual information. As we focus on reporting, it should be possible to check text on its completeness and show pop-ups when a particular field is not filled out or missing. The same is true for adding a particular classification or urgency to the report based on textual or imaging data. It is necessary to check this in an application, such as a GUI. In addition, case selection should be facilitated based on image or textual characteristics, to only send a subset of cases or specific cases to a particular AI tool. A potential user interface should be flexible enough to facilitate this.

9.6.3 Free Text vs. (Semi-)Structured Data

In the field of radiology reporting, there is an ongoing debate whether we need unstructured free text or structured reports [39, 44]. Free text will give the reporter flexibility in reporting, whereas a structured format is somewhat rigid yet contains a more reusable content. However, one important aspect of implementing NLP is the availability and usability of the data, as good standardized and structured data is conditional for the NLP tool to perform best. For now, it is too simple to think that NLP is changing the radiological reporting process at such a level, that standardization and structuring data is not necessary anymore. Especially standardization, the use of structuring tools, such as LOINC and SNOMED CT as well as the FAIR principles still need to be followed [81]. Hence, it is best to have FAIR data than to make data FAIR. For both encoding and decoding transformers, or a combination of both, standardized and structured data still perform best.

Indeed, current developments like ChatGPT show that it is possible to look beyond these boundaries and perhaps standardization and structure are becoming less important. However, keep in mind that in healthcare, and therefore in radiology practice, implementations of developments in the field of AI are being valued differently than in other fields, resulting in delayed adaptation.

9.6.4 Future

When looking into the future, it is possible to use transformers for all kinds of purposes in the reporting process. However, it is important to first focus on these applications on either the encoder or decoder end of the spectrum. When focusing on high-end applications that can be used in the orange zone, we should still focus on the purpose of the radiological report: transferring information and answering the clinical question. Hereby, the necessity of producing a proper report by means of content consistency as well as a proper structure of the final report remains highly important. The report should still be readable and accurate for the referring clinician, GP, or patient. In addition, looking into the future, the availability of (validated and structured) inputs on which the final NLP-generated radiological report is based, becomes very important. In the conventional reporting process, the radiologist reads the examination and decides, based on his or her knowledge, what should be stated in the radiological report. When using LLMs, the writing part of this process is outsourced. However, the information transfer from the image to the reporter and further to the LLM is still necessary and needs to be smooth and exact. This information process is becoming especially important as AI tools will be increasingly involved in the reporting process, supporting or partially replacing the radiologist. Both observations (1) readable and accurate radiological report and (2) how will AI interfere in the reporting process are issues we need to address in the near future.

The AI act is also very important, when we focus on legal issues. Who is responsible for the use of such tools and what difference can be made in tools supporting the radiological reporter and tools that function on their own? Do tools need to be CE-certified and/or FDA approved? Furthermore, where is the data stored, during processing: in the cloud or at a local server? This all highly depends on the type of tool, its application, the used data, and the local setting.

Ultimately, the question will be whether it is possible to make a report out of solely the interpretation of the image, by image mining or some AI image tool, without a radiologist, or whether it is still necessary that data needs to be reviewed, annotated, and structured by the reporter. To put it in a different way: who does the thinking? Indeed, it is already known that AI used for image processing can be used as input in radiology reporting, but this input is always limited to some parts of the report and is not covering the content of the whole report. In addition, when looking at the bigger picture: is it possible to integrate other diagnostics, such as pathology, laboratory results, and genetics, in the general reporting process facilitated by AI leading to more integrated diagnostics. As such, these are relevant questions of the application of LLMs, we should be aware of at this point of time and that need to be answered in upcoming years.

References

1. European Society of Radiology (ESR). Good practice for radiological reporting. Guidelines from the European Society of Radiology (ESR). Insights. Imaging. 2011;2(2):93–6. https://doi.org/10.1007/s13244-011-0066-7.

2. Grieve FM, Plumb AA, Khan SH. Radiology reporting: a general practitioner's perspective. Br J Radiol. 2010;83(985):17–22. https://doi.org/10.1259/bjr/16360063.

3. Recommandations générales pour l'élaboration d'un compte-rendu radiologique (CRR). J Radiol. 2007;88(2):304–6. https://doi.org/10.1016/S0221-0363(07)89822-2.

4. American College of Radiology. ACR practice guideline for communication of diagnostic imaging findings [internet]. Reston, VA: American College of Radiology; 2005. [cited September 2020]. https://www.acr.org/-/media/acr/files/practice-parameters/communicationdiag.pdf

5. The Royal College of Radiologists. Standards for the reporting and interpretation of imaging investigations [internet]. London: The Royal College of Radiologists; 2006. [cited September 2020]. https://www.rcr.ac.uk/sites/default/files/bfcr061_standardsforreporting.pdf

6. Wallis A, McCoubrie P. The radiology report—are we getting the message across? Clin Radiol. 2011;66(11):1015–22. https://doi.org/10.1016/j.crad.2011.05.013.

7. Berlin L. Pitfalls of the vague radiology report. AJR Am J Roentgenol. 2000;174(6):1511–8. https://doi.org/10.2214/ajr.174.6.1741511.

8. Eisenberg RL. Radiology and the law: malpractice and other issues. New York, NY: Springer; 2003.

9. Sistrom CL, Langlotz CP. A framework for improving radiology reporting. J Am Coll Radiol. 2005;2:159e67. https://doi.org/10.1016/j.jacr.2004.06.015.

10. Langlotz CP. The radiology report: a guide to thoughtful communication for radiologists and other medical professionals. CreateSpace Independent Publishing Platform; 2015.

11. Brady AP. Radiology reporting—from Hemingway to HAL? Insights Imaging. 2018;9(2):237–46. https://doi.org/10.1007/s13244-018-0596-3.

12. Weiss DL, Kim W, Branstetter BF IV, Prevedello LM. Radiology reporting: a closed-loop cycle from order entry to results communication. J Am Coll Radiol. 2014;11(12):1226–37. https://doi.org/10.1016/j.jacr.2014.09.009.

13. Joshi V, Narra VR, Joshi K, Lee K, Melson D. PACS administrators' and radiologists' perspective on the importance of features for PACS selection. J Digit Imaging. 2014;27(4):486–95. https://doi.org/10.1007/s10278-014-9682-3.

14. Geis JR. Medical imaging informatics: how it improves radiology practice today. J Digit Imaging. 2007;20(2):99–104. https://doi.org/10.1007/s10278-007-9010-2.

15. Weiss DL, Bolos PR. Reporting and dictation. In: Branstetter IV BF, editor. Practical imaging informatics: foundations and applications for PACS professionals. New York, NY: Springer; 2009. p. 147–62.

16. Creighton C. A literature review on communication between picture archiving and communication systems and radiology information sys-

tems and/or hospital information systems. J Digit Imaging. 1999;12(3):138–43. https://doi.org/10.1007/BF03168632.

17. Liu D, Zucherman M, Tulloss WB Jr. Six characteristics of effective structured reporting and the inevitable integration with speech recognition. J Digit Imaging. 2006;19:98–104. https://doi.org/10.1007/s10278-005-8734-0.

18. Glaser C, Trumm C, Nissen-Meyer S, Francke M, Küttner B, Reiser M. Spracherkennung: Auswirkung auf workflow und Befundverfügbarkeit [speech recognition: impact on workflow and report availability]. Radiologe. 2005;45(8):735–42. https://doi.org/10.1007/s00117-005-1253-7.

19. Kauppinen T, Koivikko MP, Ahovuo J. Improvement of report workflow and productivity using speech recognition—a follow-up study. J Digit Imaging. 2008;21(4):378–82. https://doi.org/10.1007/s10278-008-9121-4. Erratum in: J Digit Imaging 2008;21(4):383

20. Reiner BI. Expanding the functionality of speech recognition in radiology: creating a real-time methodology for measurement and analysis of occupational stress and fatigue. J Digit Imaging. 2013;26(1):5–9. https://doi.org/10.1007/s10278-012-9540-0.

21. Yang L, Ene IC, Arabi Belaghi R, Koff D, Stein N, Santaguida PL. Stakeholders' perspectives on the future of artificial intelligence in radiology: a scoping review. Eur Radiol. 2022;32(3):1477–95. https://doi.org/10.1007/s00330-021-08214-z. Epub 2021 Sep 21

22. Al-Naser YA. The impact of artificial intelligence on radiography as a profession: a narrative review. J Med Imaging Radiat Sci. 2023;54(1):162–6. https://doi.org/10.1016/j.jmir.2022.10.196. Epub 2022 Nov 12

23. Erickson BJ, Korfiatis P, Kline TL, Akkus Z, Philbrick K, Weston AD. Deep learning in radiology: does one size fit all? J Am Coll Radiol. 2018;15(3 Pt B):521–6. https://doi.org/10.1016/j.jacr.2017.12.027.

24. Huisman M, Ranschaert E, Parker W, Mastrodicasa D, Koci M, Pinto de Santos D, Coppola F, Morozov S, Zins M, Bohyn C, Koç U, Wu J, Veean S, Fleischmann D, Leiner T, Willemink MJ. An international survey on AI in radiology in 1041 radiologists and radiology residents part 2: expectations, hurdles to implementation, and education. Eur Radiol. 2021;31(11):8797–806. https://doi.org/10.1007/s00330-021-07782-4. Epub 2021 May 11. PMID: 33974148; PMCID: PMC8111651

25. Brady AP, Allen B, Chong J, Kotter E, Kottler N, Mongan J, Oakden-Rayner L, Dos Santos DP, Tang A, Wald C, Slavotinek J. Developing, purchasing, implementing and monitoring AI tools in radiology: practical considerations. A multi-society statement from the ACR, CAR, ESR, RANZCR & RSNA. Insights Imaging. 2024;15(1):16. https://doi.org/10.1186/s13244-023-01541-3. PMID: 38246898; PMCID: PMC10800328

26. Bizzo BC, Almeida RR, Alkasab TK. Artificial intelligence enabling radiology reporting. Radiol Clin North Am. 2021;59(6):1045–52. https://doi.org/10.1016/j.rcl.2021.07.004.

27. Monshi MMA, Poon J, Chung V. Deep learning in generating radiology reports: a survey. Artif Intell Med. 2020;106:101878. https://doi.org/10.1016/j.artmed.2020.101878. Epub 2020 May 15. PMID: 32425358; PMCID: PMC7227610

28. Lambin P, Leijenaar RTH, Deist TM, Peerlings J, de Jong EEC, van Timmeren J, et al. Radiomics: the bridge between medical imaging and personalized medicine. Nat Rev Clin Oncol. 2017;14(12):749–62. https://doi.org/10.1038/nrclinonc.2017.141.

29. Guiot J, Vaidyanathan A, Deprez L, Zerka F, Danthine D, Frix AN, et al. A review in radiomics: making personalized medicine a reality via routine imaging. Med Res Rev. 2022;42(1):426–40. https://doi.org/10.1002/med.21846.

30. Reginelli A, Nardone V, Giacobbe G, Belfiore MP, Grassi R, Schettino F, et al. Radiomics as a new frontier of imaging for cancer prognosis: a narrative review. Diagnostics. 2021;11(10):1796. https://doi.org/10.3390/diagnostics11101796.

31. van Leeuwen KG, Schalekamp S, Rutten MJCM, van Ginneken B, de Rooij M. Artificial intelligence in radiology: 100 commercially available products and their scientific evidence. Eur Radiol. 2021;31(6):3797–804. https://doi.org/10.1007/s00330-021-07892-z. Epub 2021 Apr 15. PMID: 33856519; PMCID: PMC8128724

32. Reiner BI, Knight N, Siegel EL. Radiology reporting, past, present, and future: the radiologist's perspective. J Am Coll Radiol. 2007;4(5):313–9. https://doi.org/10.1016/j.jacr.2007.01.015.

33. European Society of Radiology (ESR). ESR concept paper on value-based radiology. Insights Imaging. 2017;8(5):447–54. https://doi.org/10.1007/s13244-017-0566-1.

34. Kahn CE Jr, Langlotz CP, Burnside ES, Carrino JA, Channin DS, Hovsepian DM, et al. Toward best practices in radiology reporting. Radiology. 2009;252(3):852–6. https://doi.org/10.1148/radiol.2523081992.

35. Lukaszewicz A, Uricchio J, Gerasymchuk G. The art of the radiology report: practical and stylistic guidelines for perfecting the conveyance of imaging findings. Can Assoc Radiol J. 2016;67(4):318–21. https://doi.org/10.1016/j.carj.2016.03.001.

36. Reiner BI. The challenges, opportunities, and imperative of structured reporting in medical imaging. J Digit Imaging. 2009;22(6):562–8. https://doi.org/10.1007/s10278-009-9239-z.

37. Hall FM. Language of the radiology report: primer for residents and wayward radiologists. AJR Am J Roentgenol. 2000;175(5):1239–42. https://doi.org/10.2214/ajr.175.5.1751239.

38. Jacoby J, Ayer R. Frameworks for radiology reporting. London: Taylor and Francis; 2009.

39. European Society of Radiology (ESR). ESR paper on structured reporting in radiology. Insights Imaging. 2018;9(1):1–7. https://doi.org/10.1007/s13244-017-0588-8.
40. Fatehi M. In: dos Santos DP, editor. Structured reporting in radiology. Springer; 2022.
41. Nobel JM, Kok EM, Robben SGF. Redefining the structure of structured reporting in radiology. Insights Imaging. 2020;11(1):10. https://doi.org/10.1186/s13244-019-0831-6.
42. An JY, Unsdorfer KML, Weinreb JC. BI-RADS, C-RADS, CAD-RADS, LI-RADS, Lung-RADS, NI-RADS, O-RADS, PI-RADS, TI-RADS: reporting and data systems. Radiographics. 2019;39(5):1435–6. https://doi.org/10.1148/rg.2019190087.
43. Radiological Society of North America. RadReport template library [Internet]. Oak Brook, IL: Radiological Society of North America; 2020. [cited 15 Dec 2020]. https://radreport.org
44. European Society of Radiology (ESR). ESR paper on structured reporting in radiology-update 2023. Insights Imaging. 2023;14(1):199. https://doi.org/10.1186/s13244-023-01560-0.
45. Wilkinson MD, Dumontier M, Aalbersberg IJ, Appleton G, Axton M, Baak A, et al. The FAIR guiding principles for scientific data management and stewardship. Sci Data. 2016;3:160018. https://doi.org/10.1038/sdata.2016.18. Erratum in: Sci Data 2019;6(1):6
46. Kreimeyer K, Foster M, Pandey A, Arya N, Halford G, Jones SF, et al. Natural language processing systems for capturing and standardizing unstructured clinical information: a systematic review. J Biomed Inform. 2017;73:14–29. https://doi.org/10.1016/j.jbi.2017.07.012.
47. Pinto Dos Santos D, Baeßler B. Big data, artificial intelligence, and structured reporting. Eur Radiol Exp. 2018;2(1):42. https://doi.org/10.1186/s41747-018-0071-4.
48. Mozayan A, Fabbri AR, Maneevese M, Tocino I, Chheang S. Practical guide to natural language processing for radiology. Radiographics. 2021;41(5):1446–53. https://doi.org/10.1148/rg.2021200113.
49. Smyth P. Data mining: data analysis on a grand scale? Stat Methods Med Res. 2000;9(4):309–27. https://doi.org/10.1177/096228020000900402.
50. Pons E, Braun LMM, Hunink MGM, Kors JA. Natural language processing in radiology: a systematic review. Radiology. 2016;279:329–43. https://doi.org/10.1148/radiol.16142770.
51. Cáceres SB. Electronic health records: beyond the digitization of medical files. Clinics. 2013;68(8):1077–8. https://doi.org/10.6061/clinics/2013(08)02.
52. Elkassem AA, Smith AD. Potential use cases for ChatGPT in radiology reporting. AJR Am J Roentgenol. 2023;221(3):373–6. https://doi.org/10.2214/AJR.23.29198. Epub 2023 Apr 19
53. Lecler A, Duron L, Soyer P. Revolutionizing radiology with GPT-based models: current applications, future possibilities and limitations of

ChatGPT. Diagn Interv Imaging. 2023;104(6):269–74. https://doi.org/10.1016/j.diii.2023.02.003. Epub 2023 Feb 28

54. Bajaj S, Gandhi D, Nayar D. Potential applications and impact of ChatGPT in radiology. Acad Radiol. 2024;31:1256–61. https://doi.org/10.1016/j.acra.2023.08.039. Epub ahead of print

55. Dave T, Athaluri SA, Singh S. ChatGPT in medicine: an overview of its applications, advantages, limitations, future prospects, and ethical considerations. Front Artif Intell. 2023;6:1169595. https://doi.org/10.3389/frai.2023.1169595.

56. Locke S, Bashall A, Al-Adely S, Moore J, Wilson A, Kitchen GB. Natural language processing in medicine: a review. Trends Anaesth Crit Care. 2021;38:4–9.

57. Misha BK, Kumar R. Natural language processing in artificial intelligence. 1st ed. Apple Academic; 2020.

58. Thirunavukarasu AJ, Ting DSJ, Elangovan K, Gutierrez L, Tan TF, Ting DSW. Large language models in medicine. Nat Med. 2023;29(8):1930–40. https://doi.org/10.1038/s41591-023-02448-8.

59. Tunstall L, von Werra L, Wolf T. Natural language processing with transformers. 1st ed. O'Reilly Media, Inc; 2022.

60. Meskó B. The impact of multimodal large language models on health care's future. J Med Internet Res. 2023;25:e52865. https://doi.org/10.2196/52865. PMID: 37917126; PMCID: PMC10654899

61. Qi S, Cao Z, Rao J, Wang L, Xiao J, Wang X. What is the limitation of multimodal LLMs? A deeper look into multimodal LLMs through prompt probing. Inf Process Manag. 2023;60(6):103510.,ISSN 0306-4573. https://doi.org/10.1016/j.ipm.2023.103510.

62. Hansell DM, Bankier AA, MacMahon H, McLoud TC, Müller NL, Remy J. Fleischner society: glossary of terms for thoracic imaging. Radiology. 2008;246(3):697–722. https://doi.org/10.1148/radiol.2462070712.

63. Pham AD, Névéol A, Lavergne T, et al. Natural language processing of radiology reports for the detection of thromboembolic diseases and clinically relevant incidental findings. BMC Bioinformatics. 2014;15:266. https://doi.org/10.1186/1471-2105-15-266.

64. Rink B, Roberts K, Harabagiu S, et al. Extracting actionable findings of appendicitis from radiology reports using natural language processing. AMIA Jt Summits Transl Sci Proc. 2013;2013:221.

65. Mendonça EA, Haas J, Shagina L, Larson E, Friedman C. Extracting information on pneumonia in infants using natural language processing of radiology reports. J Biomed Inform. 2005;38(4):314–21. https://doi.org/10.1016/j.jbi.2005.02.003.

66. Haas JP, Mendonça EA, Ross B, Friedman C, Larson E. Use of computerized surveillance to detect nosocomial pneumonia in neonatal intensive care unit patients. Am J Infect Control. 2005;33(8):439–43. https://doi.org/10.1016/j.ajic.2005.06.008.

67. Do BH, Wu AS, Maley J, Biswal S. Automatic retrieval of bone fracture knowledge using natural language processing. J Digit Imaging. 2013;26(4):709–13. https://doi.org/10.1007/s10278-012-9531-1.
68. Fiszman M, Chapman WW, Aronsky D, Evans RS, Haug PJ. Automatic detection of acute bacterial pneumonia from chest x-ray reports. J Am Med Inform Assoc. 2000;7(6):593–604. https://doi.org/10.1136/jamia.2000.0070593.
69. Fiszman M, Chapman WW, Evans SR, Haug PJ. Automatic identification of pneumonia related concepts on chest x-ray reports. Proc AMIA Symp. 1999;7–71
70. Yim WW, Yetisgen M, Harris WP, Kwan SW. Natural language processing in oncology: a review. JAMA Oncol. 2016;2(6):797–804. https://doi.org/10.1001/jamaoncol.2016.0213.
71. Lee SJ, Weinberg BD, Gore A, Banerjee I. A scalable natural language processing for inferring BTRADS categorization from unstructured brain magnetic resonance reports. J Digit Imaging. 2020;33(6):1393–400. https://doi.org/10.1007/s10278-020-00350-0.
72. Zeng Z, Espino S, Roy A, Li X, Khan SA, Clare SE, et al. Using natural language processing and machine learning to identify breast cancer local recurrence. BMC Bioinformatics. 2018;19(Suppl 17):498. https://doi.org/10.1186/s12859-018-2466-x.
73. Lou R, Lalevic D, Chambers C, Zafar HM, Cook TS. Automated detection of radiology reports that require follow-up imaging using natural language processing feature engineering and machine learning classification. J Digit Imaging. 2020;33(1):131–6. https://doi.org/10.1007/s10278-019-00271-7.6.
74. Abdulsalam AKAAI, Garvin JH, Redd A, Carter ME, Sweeny C, Meystre SM. Automated extraction and classification of cancer stage mentions from unstructured text fields in a central cancer registry. AMIA Jt Summits Transl Sci Proc. 2017;2018:16–25.
75. Kehl KL, Elmarakeby H, Nishino M, Van Allen EM, Lepisto EM, Hassett MJ, et al. Assessment of dee7p natural language processing in ascertaining oncologic outcomes from radiology reports. JAMA Oncol. 2019;5(10):1421–9. https://doi.org/10.1001/jamaoncol.2019.1800.
76. Cheng LT, Zheng J, Savova GK, Erickson BJ. Discerning tumor status from unstructured MRI reports: completeness of information in existing reports and utility of automated natural language processing. J Digit Imaging. 2010;23(2):119–32. https://doi.org/10.1007/s10278-009-9215-7.
77. Jain NL, Friedman C. Identification of findings suspicious for breast cancer based on natural language processing of mammogram reports. Proc AMIA Annu Fall Symp. 1997;829–833
78. Percha B, Nassif H, Lipson J, Burnside E, Rubin D. Automatic classification of mammography reports by BI-RADS breast tissue composition class. J Am Med Inform Assoc. 2012;19(5):913–6. https://doi.org/10.1136/amiajnl-2011-000607.

79. Singhal K, Azizi S, Tu T, Mahdavi SS, Wei J, Chung HW, Scales N, Tanwani A, Cole-Lewis H, Pfohl S, Payne P, Seneviratne M, Gamble P, Kelly C, Babiker A, Schärli N, Chowdhery A, Mansfield P, Demner-Fushman D, Agüera Y, Arcas B, Webster D, Corrado GS, Matias Y, Chou K, Gottweis J, Tomasev N, Liu Y, Rajkomar A, Barral J, Semturs C, Karthikesalingam A, Natarajan V. Large language models encode clinical knowledge. Nature. 2023;620(7972):172–80. https://doi.org/10.1038/s41586-023-06291-2. Epub 2023 Jul 12. Erratum in: Nature. 2023 Jul 27;: PMID: 37438534; PMCID: PMC10396962

80. Perera Molligoda Arachchige AS. Empowering radiology: the transformative role of ChatGPT. Clin Radiol. 2023;78(11):851–5. https://doi.org/10.1016/j.crad.2023.08.006. Epub 2023 Aug 22

81. Wang KC. Standard lexicons, coding systems and ontologies for interoperability and semantic computation in imaging. J Digit Imaging. 2018;31(3):353–60. https://doi.org/10.1007/s10278-018-0069-8. PMID: 29725962; PMCID: PMC5959830